Glycolysis

Krebs cycle

β Oxidation

Respiratory chain

Cytosol

Mitochondrion

matrix
inner membrane
intermembrane space
outer membrane

Metabolism at a Glance

J.G. Salway

Associate Senior Lecturer in Medical Biochemistry
School of Biomedical and Molecular Sciences
University of Surrey
Guildford, UK
j.salway@btinternet.com

FOREWORD BY
D.K. Granner
Vanderbilt University Medical Center
Nashville, USA

THIRD EDITION

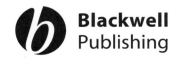
Blackwell
Publishing

© 2004 by Blackwell Publishing Ltd
Blackwell Publishing, Inc., 350 Main Street, Malden, Massachusetts 02148-5020, USA
Blackwell Publishing Ltd, 9600 Garsington Road, Oxford OX4 2DQ, UK
Blackwell Publishing Asia Pty Ltd, 550 Swanston Street, Carlton, Victoria 3053, Australia

First published 1994
First Japanese edition 1994
Reprinted 1995, 1996, 1998
Second edition 1999
Reprinted 2000, 2002, 2003
Second Japanese edition 2000
German edition 2000
Spanish edition 2002
Third edition 2004

ISBN 1-4051-0716-2

Catalogue records for this title are available from the British Library and Library of Congress

Set in 9¼ pt Times by Oxford Designers & Illustrators, Oxford
Printed and bound in Italy by G. Canale & C. SpA, Turin

Commissioning Editor: Vicki Noyes
Managing Editor: Geraldine Jeffers
Production Editor: Jonathan Rowley
Production Controller: Kate Charman

For further information on Blackwell Publishing, visit our website:
http://www.blackwellpublishing.com

Contents

Foreword

Our forebears must have marvelled at how food and drink somehow sustained life. As science slowly evolved over the millenia it surely became apparent that Nature, when understood, has a special beauty and symmetry. This is nowhere more apparent than in the observation that one can now trace the metabolic fate of a certain substrate through numerous interrelated and carefully controlled pathways to its ultimate destination, the biologic equivalent of a global positioning system. The information base that enables one to take this journey certainly represents one of the great accomplishments of 20th century biological science. The study of metabolism reached its zenith one or two generations ago when scholars purified and characterized hundreds of enzymes using techniques so tedious, inefficient and sometimes dangerous that current students and scientists have difficulty believing these procedures even existed. The substrates and products of these enzymatic reactions were systematically defined, as were a variety of regulatory mechanisms that control the flux through the various pathways. It all seems so logical and straightforward now, but imagine the confusion that existed as the individual bits of data were presented and before enough was known to assemble the first 'metabolic chart.'

The study of metabolism has, perhaps, been eclipsed by other fields of endeavour that certainly attract more attention from students and investigators, better notice in the lay and scientific press and favoured research funding. This point was driven home to me a few years ago when I went searching for a metabolic chart for the purpose of making a series of introductory slides for a lecture. I conducted my own version of a futile cycle through numerous offices and laboratories in the vain quest. I saw many charts of oncogenes, signal transduction pathways and the organization of the marine and human genomes, but none of the metabolic pathway. Finally, a postdoctoral fellow came to the rescue when he recalled that he had a metabolic chart rolled up in a tube in a closet in his apartment.

Those who continue to explore the mysteries of metabolism, and new pieces of the puzzle are still being located and placed, lament a perceived lack of interest in the topic by students and young scientists and teachers. They (we) imagine that the inherent beauty of the system should suffice to attract attention. But science moves forward because new areas of interest are defined and novel ways of exploring these topics are developed. New and unexplored terrain is always enticing, particularly to the young who are blessed with the neuronal plasticity necessary for rapid adaptation. In spite of the dire prediction that the advent of molecular biology heralded the end of serious science (a view shared by many physiologists and students of metabolism) quite the opposite has happened. Novel experimental techniques have led to the precise definition of the DNA mutations responsible for more than 2000 human genetic diseases, and at least another 12 000 genes are likely to be associated with various maladies. The phenotypic manifestations of many of these mutations can only be understood through knowledge of metabolic pathways. The stunning ability to alter the genome of experimental animals by transgenic and gene knockout technology has led to the appearance of phenotypes that the molecular biologist often cannot predict in advance, or begin to explain after the fact. This has resulted, inevitably, in a resurgent need for people who understand metabolism. It is often difficult to find qualified senior collaborators in this area, and the supply pipeline is not bursting with young replacements. One reason for this is that, regrettably, this topic is not taught well at many institutions, if it is taught at all. It certainly is rare, in the US at least, to encounter an entering graduate student who has taken an undergraduate course in metabolism. Not unusual is the student well versed in immunology, molecular biology, oncology, neurobiology and genetics, to name a few subjects. There are, no doubt, several explanations for this, and not the least of these is the way the subject is taught. I suspect students asked to give a first response to the question 'What do you think of when you hear the word metabolism?' would quickly respond 'impenetrable charts'. The subject has not always been presented in a clear, exciting and relevant way in textbooks or classrooms. *Metabolism at a Glance* represents a career-long effort by J.G. Salway to make the subject of metabolism approachable, interesting and relevant to human disease. The book is successful on all accounts, and plays an important role as a supplemental text for students, and as a reference source for scientists and teachers. It is a mainstay in my laboratory.

Many books, including textbooks, never get past the first edition. The fact that a third edition of *Metabolism At a Glance* is warranted is indeed an accomplishment. This bespeaks the point that metabolism is still a dynamic field and that Dr Salway's approach to the subject is on target. His effort is helping restore this discipline to the position it so richly deserves.

One final point, I hope to see the day when someone like George Lucas (LucasFilms) uses a 'Star Wars' cinematic approach to devise a tour through a four-dimensional, integrated representation of the metabolic, signal transduction and gene regulation pathways, perhaps as an interactive computer game. Imagine yourself starting as a glucose molecule starting on this journey. This is a trip that will attract people's attention and interest!

D.K. Granner
Vanderbilt Diabetes Center
Vanderbilt University Medical Center
Nashville, TN
USA

May 2003

Preface

The 'At a Glance' format of two-page spreads for each topic imposes on the author the discipline of brevity. The dilemma is the need for space to add new information while being reluctant to create space by removing essential text. This third edition includes new chapters on the regulation of glycolysis and the pentose phosphate pathway, and the section on diabetes has been expanded. Two new chapters have acknowledged the importance of tryptophan and tyrosine metabolism as precursors of neurologically active amines and other products. Reye's syndrome is a very rare disease now that children are not given aspirin and this is a triumph of medical education. However, its inclusion is justified because it dramatically illustrates the mutual dependence of the several metabolic pathways that operate in liver during fasting. Also, a chapter has been included on the important (but chronically neglected) subject of 'substrate channelling', which should underpin the way we think of metabolic pathways. Although there is an excellent monograph on this subject by Agius and Sherratt (see Chapter 34), it has not previously been included in a basic textbook to the knowledge of the author.

The format allows the book to be used by students of medicine, veterinary science and the biomedical sciences. It will also serve postgraduates, researchers and practising specialists in the fields of diabetes, metabolic disorders, chemical pathology and sports science. However, readers new to biochemistry will need to cherry-pick the information appropriate to their level of study with guidance from their course notes. Finally, to those who say that metabolism is hopelessly complicated: the important thing is not to be overwhelmed by information but to treat metabolic maps just as you would any road map or plan of the underground rail network and simply select the information needed for your specific purpose.

Acknowledgements

I am grateful to readers who have sent encouraging e-mails and to those who have taken the trouble to indicate errors, omissions and make suggestions. These include Professor Richard Hanson, who made half a dozen valuable suggestions that I have incorporated. Also, Dr Ann Saada (Reisch) has been a frequent correspondent who has made several important contributions. As in previous editions I have depended on subject experts for advice and guidance and I am especially grateful to the following for their help: Professor Loranne Agius, Professor Dario Alessi, Professor Jo Arendt, Dr Abdulla Badawy, Professor Ron Chalmers, Professor Sir Philip Cohen, Professor Raafat El-Maghrabi, Professor Keith Frayn, Dr Anna Gloyn, Professor Gwyn Gould, Dr Anne Green, Gordon Hartman, Dr Ron Hubbard, Professor Mitchell Lazar, Kate Monnery, Professor Debra Skene, Dr Keith Snell and Dr Malcolm von Schantz. It has been a great pleasure to collaborate with Elaine Leggett of Oxford Designers and Illustrators whose skill and enduring patience made short work of the complex metabolic charts and diagrams. Once again I am especially grateful to Rosemary James who has been a staunch supporter and source of encouragement. She has read the manuscript and her patience and attention to detail in checking for errors, ambiguities and her many contributions are much appreciated. Philip Aslett compiled the comprehensive index. As readers can imagine, this is a challenging book to produce and I am most grateful for the tolerance and support provided by Blackwell, especially Fiona Goodgame, Vicki Noyes, Geraldine Jeffers, Jonathan Rowley and Karen Moore.

Finally, despite all the care that has been taken to eliminate errors, regrettably it is inevitable that some will have slipped through the net and as always I would appreciate hearing from readers who spot any mistakes I have overlooked.

J.G. Salway

j.salway@btinternet.com

September 2003

Further reading

Devlin T.M. (ed.) (2002) *Textbook of Biochemistry with Clinical Correlations*, 5th edn. Wiley-Liss, New York.

Frayn K.N. (2003) *Metabolic Regulation: A Human Perspective*. Blackwell Publishing, Oxford.

Murray R.K., Granner D.K., Mayes P.A. & Rodwell V.W. (1999) *Harper's Biochemistry*, 25th edn. McGraw-Hill Education.

Introduction to metabolic pathways

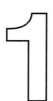

Metabolic charts

The metabolic map opposite will, at first sight, appear to most readers to be a confusing, incomprehensible jumble of chemical formulae. There can be no doubt that metabolic charts **are** complex, and many biochemists remember their own first introduction to metabolism as a somewhat bewildering experience.

The first important thing to remember is that the chart is no more than a form of map. In many respects it is similar to a map of the London Underground, which is also very complicated (see Diagram 1.1 below). With the latter, however, we have learned to suppress the overwhelming detail in order to concentrate on those aspects relevant to a particular journey. For example, if asked 'How would you get from Archway to Queensway?' the reply is likely to be: 'Take the Northern Line travelling south to Tottenham Court Road, then change to the Central Line travelling west to Queensway'. An equally valid answer would be: 'Enter Archway station, buy a ticket at the kiosk, pass through the ticket inspector's barrier and proceed to the platform. When a train arrives, enter and remain seated as it passes through Tuffnell Park, Kentish Town, Camden Town, Euston, Warren Street and Goodge Street. When it reaches Tottenham Court Road, stand up and leave the train, transfer to platform 1, etc., etc.' Each of these details, although essential for completion of the journey, is not necessary to an **overall** understanding of the journey.

A similar approach should be used when studying the metabolic chart. The details of individual enzyme reactions are very complex and very important. Many biochemists, including some of the world's most famous, have been researching individual enzymes such as **phosphofructokinase-1**, **pyruvate dehydrogenase** and **glucokinase** for many years. The detailed properties of these important enzymes and the mechanism of their reactions are superbly summarized in several standard biochemistry textbooks. However, these details should not be allowed to confuse the mind of the reader when asked the question: 'How is glucose metabolized to fat?' When faced with such a problem, the student should learn to recall sufficient detail relevant to an overall understanding of the pathways involved, while maintaining an awareness of the detailed background information and mechanisms.

Chart 1.1: Subcellular distribution of metabolic pathways

The metabolic chart opposite shows how certain pathways are located in the **cytosol** of the cell, whereas others are located in the **mitochondrion**. Certain other enzymes are associated with subcellular structures such as the **endoplasmic reticulum**, for example **glucose 6-phosphatase**. Others are associated with organelles such as the nucleus and peroxisomes which, for simplicity, are not shown in the chart.

The enzymes required to catalyse the reactions in the various metabolic pathways are organized among the different subcellular compartments within the cell. For example, the enzymes involved in **fatty acid synthesis**, the **pentose phosphate pathway** and **glycolysis** are nearly all located in the **cytosol**. As we can see, most of the reactions involved in harnessing energy for the cell, **Krebs cycle**, **β-oxidation** and **respiratory chain**, are located in the **mitochondrion**, which is frequently called 'the power house of the cell'.

Mitochondrion (plural, mitochondria)

Most animal and plant cells contain mitochondria. An important exception in most animal species is the mature red blood cell. Mitochondria are usually sausage-shaped organelles. They are surrounded by a double system of membranes conveniently described as the **outer membrane** and the **inner membrane**, which separate an **intermembrane space**. Interestingly, they contain ribosomes for protein synthesis plus some of their own genes, and reproduce by binary fission. In short, they are largely autonomous and biologists have suggested that they were originally bacterial cells that evolved a symbiotic relationship with a larger cell. They have therefore been described as 'cells within a cell'.

The outer membrane of the mitochondrion is fairly typical of most cell membranes, being composed of 50% protein and 50% lipids. It contains a channel-forming protein called **porin**, which renders it permeable to molecules of less than 10 kDa. This is in contrast to the inner membrane, which forms one of the most impermeable barriers within the cell. This inner membrane contains 80% protein and 20% lipid, and is folded inwards to form cristae (not shown), which project into the matrix. It is, however, permeable to water and gases such as oxygen. Also, certain metabolites can cross the inner membrane, but only when assisted by carrier systems such as the **dicarboxylate carrier**.

When sections of the inner membrane are stained for electron microscopy, mushroom-like projections, the F_o/F_1 **particles** appear. These are respiratory particles that are thought to be embedded in the membrane *in vivo*, but following oxidation project into the matrix. These particles are involved in **adenosine triphosphate (ATP)** synthesis by oxidative phosphorylation, and are functionally associated with the respiratory chain.

The **matrix** of the mitochondrion contains the enzymes of the **β-oxidation** pathway and also most of the enzymes needed for **Krebs cycle**. An important exception is **succinate dehydrogenase**, which is linked to the **respiratory chain** in the inner membrane. Certain mitochondria have special enzymes, for example, liver mitochondria contain the enzymes necessary for ketogenesis (see Chapter 27) and urea synthesis (see Chapter 33).

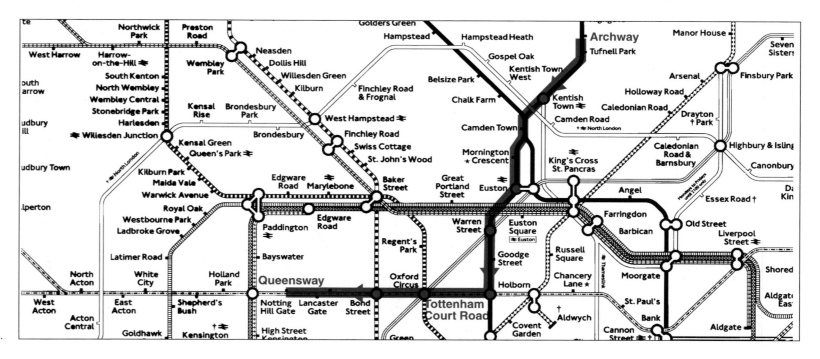

Diagram 1.1 Map of the London Underground with permission. ...red User No. 03/3954.

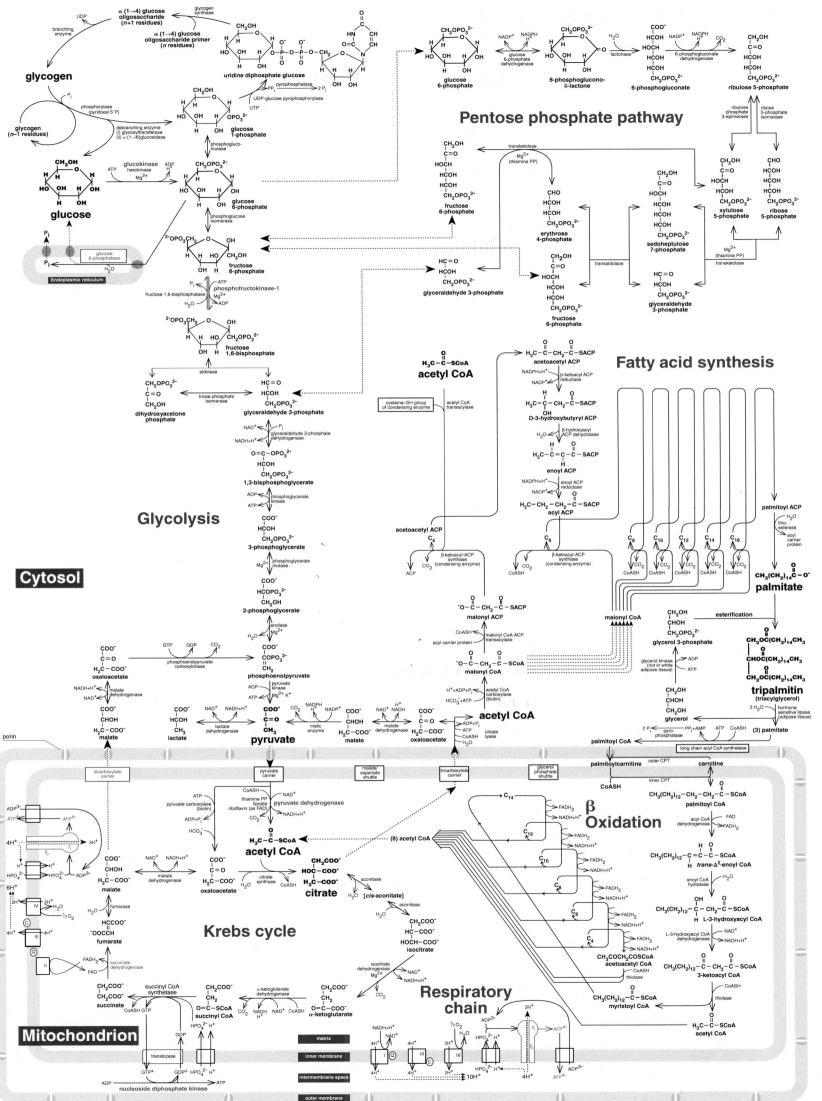

Chart 1.1 Map of the main pathways of intermediary metabolism.

Biosynthesis of ATP I: ATP, the molecule that powers metabolism

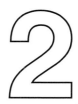

How living cells conserve energy in a biologically useful form

A lump of coal can be burned in a power station to generate electricity, which is a very useful and versatile form of energy. Apart from coal, several other fuels, such as oil, peat and even public refuse can be used to generate electricity. This electrical energy can then be used to power innumerable industrial machines and domestic appliances, which are essential to our modern way of life.

Living cells have a similarly versatile energy resource in the molecule, adenosine triphosphate (**ATP**). ATP can be generated by oxidizing several metabolic fuels, although carbohydrates and fats are especially important. ATP is used in innumerable vital metabolic reactions and physiological functions, not only in humans, but in all forms of life. The primary objective of intermediary metabolism is to maintain a steady supply of ATP so that living cells can grow, reproduce, and respond to the stresses and strains imposed by starvation, exercise, overeating, etc.

Chart 2.1: The biosynthesis of ATP

We will see later (Chapter 5) how glucose is oxidized and energy is conserved as ATP. ATP can be synthesized by phosphorylation of adenosine diphosphate (ADP) by two types of process. One does not need oxygen and is known as **substrate-level phosphorylation**. The other requires oxygen and is known as **oxidative phosphorylation**.

Substrate-level phosphorylation

Examination of the chart opposite shows that two reactions in glycolysis, namely the **phosphoglycerate kinase** and **pyruvate kinase** reactions, produce ATP by direct phosphorylation of ADP. This is **substrate-level phosphorylation** and is especially important for generating ATP if the tissues are inadequately supplied with oxygen.

ATP can also be made anaerobically from the phosphagen **phospho-creatine**, see Chapter 22.

Another example of substrate-level phosphorylation occurs in Krebs cycle. The reaction (see Diagram 2.1), catalysed by succinyl CoA synthetase, produces GTP (guanosine triphosphate), which is structurally similar to ATP. The enzyme nucleoside diphosphate kinase catalyses the conversion of GTP to ATP in the intermembrane space. **NB:** One proton is needed to transport one phosphate anion into the matrix in a process coupled to the import of GDP (guanosine diphosphate) (see Diagram 2.1).

Oxidative phosphorylation

In the presence of oxygen, oxidative phosphorylation is by far the most important mechanism for synthesizing ATP. This process is coupled to the oxidation of the reduced 'hydrogen carriers' **NADH** and **FADH$_2$** via the respiratory chain.

The 'hydrogen carriers' NAD$^+$ and FAD
NAD$^+$ (nicotinamide adenine dinucleotide)

NAD$^+$ is a hydrogen carrier derived from the vitamin niacin. It is a coenzyme involved in several oxidation/reduction reactions catalysed by dehydrogenases. In the example opposite, taken from Krebs cycle, **malate dehydrogenase** catalyses the oxidation of malate to oxaloacetate. During this reaction, NAD$^+$ is reduced to form NADH, which is oxidized by the respiratory chain and 2.5 molecules of ATP are formed (see Chapter 6).

FAD (flavin adenine dinucleotide)

FAD is a hydrogen carrier derived from the vitamin riboflavin. It differs from NAD$^+$ in that it is covalently bound to its dehydrogenase enzyme, and is therefore known as a prosthetic group. In the example opposite the **succinate dehydrogenase** reaction is shown with FAD being reduced to FADH$_2$. Succinate dehydrogenase is bound to the inner membrane of the mitochondrion and is an integral part of the respiratory chain. When FADH$_2$ is oxidized by this process, a total of 1.5 ATP molecules are formed (see Chapter 6).

ATP/ADP translocase

The inner membrane of the mitochondrion is impermeable to ATP. A protein complex known as the ATP/ADP translocase is needed for the export of ATP in return for the import of ADP (adenosine diphosphate) and phosphate anion.

The ATP molecule has two phosphoanhydride bonds that provide the energy for life

The ATP molecule has two phosphoanhydride bonds that, when hydrolysed at physiological pH, release 7.3 kcal (30.66 kJ) as energy, which can be used for metabolic purposes. These two phosphoanhydride bonds were referred to by Lipmann in 1941 as 'high-energy' bonds. However, this term is a misleading concept that (apologies apart) has been banished from the textbooks. In fact, these phosphoanhydride bonds are no different from any other covalent bonds.

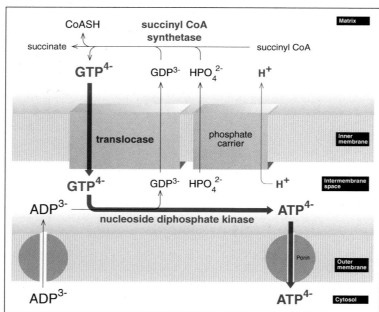

Diagram 2.2 Adenosine triphosphate.

Reference

Carusi E.A. (1992) It's time we replaced 'high-energy phosphate group' with 'phosphoryl group'. *Biochem Ed*, **20**, 145–7.

Diagram 2.1 GTP formed in the mitochondrial matrix by substrate level phosphorylation is used to form ATP in the intermembrane space for export to the cytosol.

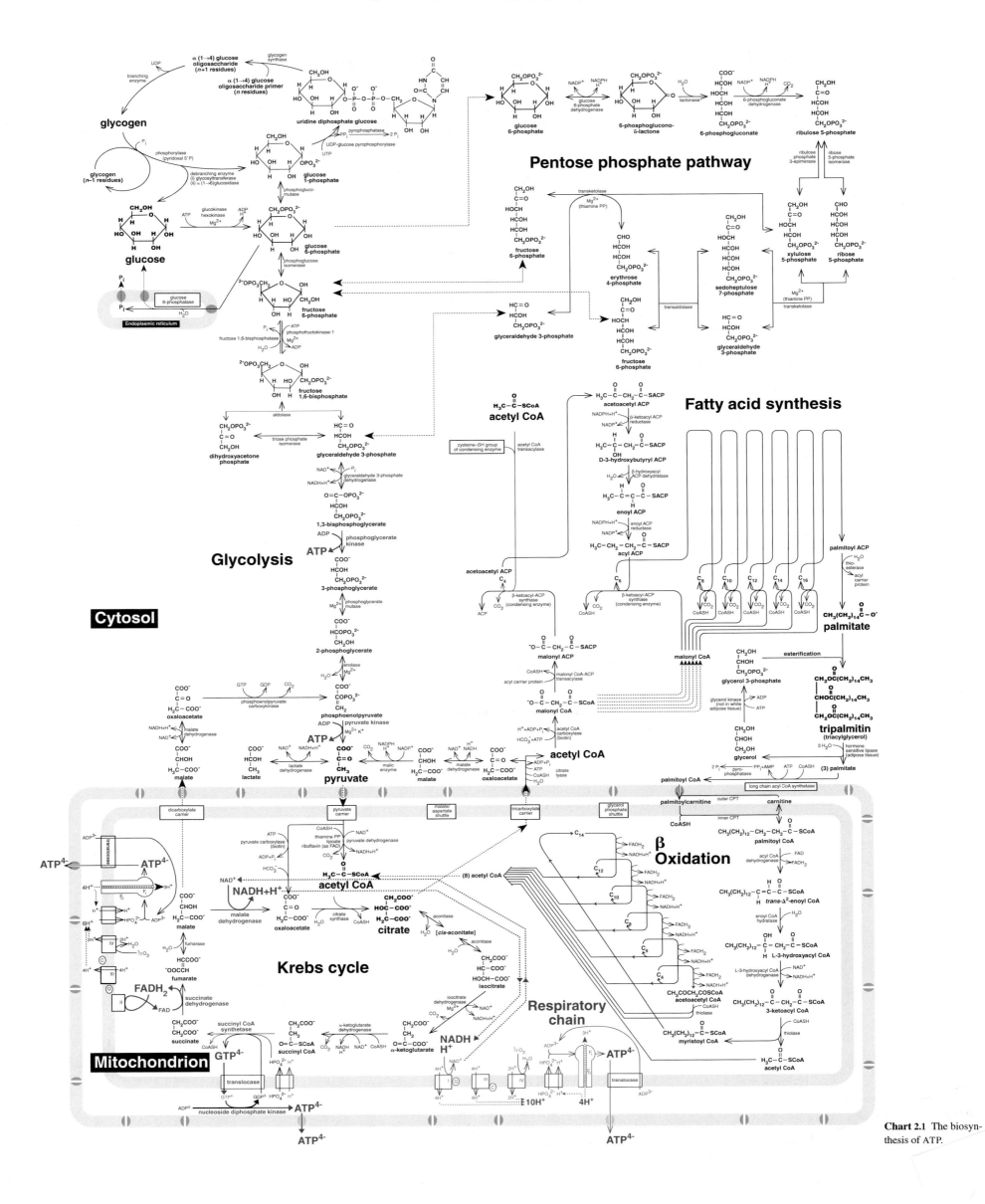

Chart 2.1 The biosynthesis of ATP.

Biosynthesis of ATP II: mitochondrial respiratory chain

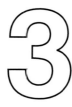

Don't panic! At a first reading, students should use the simplified diagrams 3.1a and 3.1b. Diagram 3.2 provides a more detailed summary for advanced students.

The mitochondrial respiratory chain (see Diagrams 3.1a and 3.1b) comprises a series of reduction/oxidation reactions within complexes I, II, III, and IV. These are linked by ubiquinone (Q) and cytochrome c (cytc). Ubiquinone (Q), which accepts electrons and protons as it is reduced to ubiquinol (QH₂), shuttles from both complexes I and II, to complex III. Similarly, cytochrome c shuttles electrons from complex III to complex IV. The synthesis of ATP via the respiratory chain is the result of two coupled processes: **(i) electron transport**; and **(ii) oxidative phosphorylation**.

(i) Electron transport (Diagram 3.1a). This involves the oxidation (i.e. the removal of electrons) from NADH, or FADH₂, with transport of the electrons through a chain of oxidation/reduction reactions involving cytochromes until they are donated to molecular oxygen, which is consequently reduced to water.

(ii) Oxidative phosphorylation and proton transport (Diagram 3.1b).

According to Mitchell's Chemiosmotic Theory, the electron transport just described drives proton pumps in complexes I, III and IV by a mechanism which is still not fully understood. Positively charged protons are pumped out of the mitochondrial matrix but **not** with any associated negatively charged anions. Consequently, as a result of this **charge separation**, the matrix side of the membrane becomes negatively charged, whilst the extruded protons ensure that its opposite side becomes positively charged. The difference in electrochemical potential across the membrane, which is 8 nm thick, is about 150–250 mV. This may seem unremarkable but is equivalent to 250 000 V/cm! It is this potential difference that provides the energy for ATP synthesis when the protons return to the matrix through the F₀ proton channel, thereby driving the F₁ ATP synthetase.

Proton extrusion

Although still controversial, it is assumed here that the transport of two electrons enables complex I and III each to extrude **4** H⁺, while complex IV pumps **2** H⁺.

Diagram 3.1a Electron transport. The respiratory chain showing the flow of electrons from NADH and FADH₂ to oxygen with the formation of water. NB Ascorbate (vitamin C) and TMPD are **experimental** donors/acceptors which are used in studies of mitochondria *in vitro*.

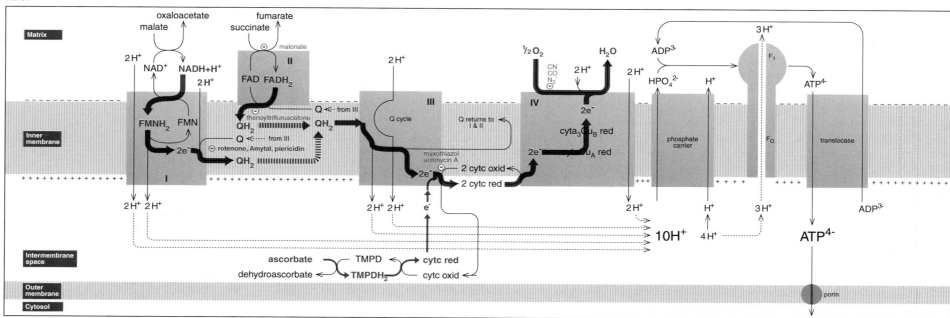

Diagram 3.1b Proton flow. The respiratory chain showing the extrusion of protons by complexes I, III and IV creating an electro-chemical gradient. As the protons return through the ATP synthetase complex, ADP is phosphorylated to ATP.

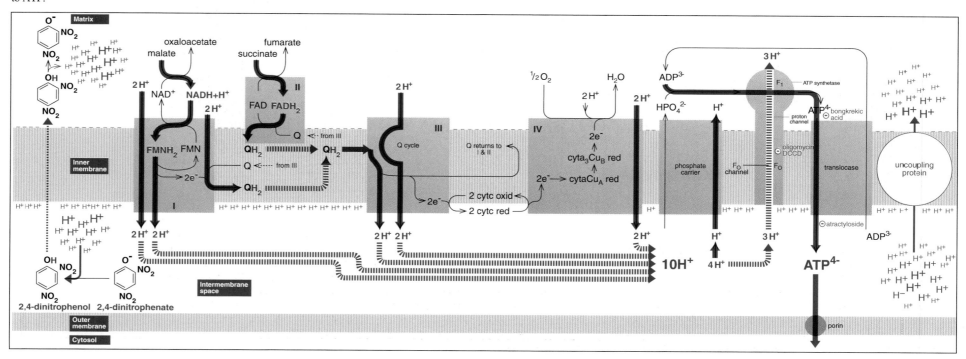

Stoichiometry of ATP synthesis

Current consensus opinion is that 3 H^+ are needed to form 1 ATP molecule, and an additional H^+ is needed to translocate it to the cytosol, i.e. a total of 4 H^+ per ATP synthesized.

P/O ratios: 'traditional' integral and 'modern' non-integral values

The number of molecules of ATP synthesized per molecule of oxygen consumed has traditionally been accepted as integral values, i.e. 3 for NADH; and 2 for $FADH_2$. However, current opinion challenges this assumption. Diagram 3.1b shows that when NADH is oxidized, a total of 10 H^+ are extruded. Since 4 H^+ are needed to make 1 ATP, oxidation of NADH yields the equivalent of 2.5 ATP molecules (i.e. the P/O ratio is the non-integral value 2.5). Similarly, for $FADH_2$, the P/O ratio is 1.5 (see Chapter 6).

Inhibitors of the respiratory chain

Compounds that inhibit or interact with Keilin's respiratory chain (pronounced 'Kaylin') have contributed to our understanding of this process. These compounds (see Diagrams 3.1a and 3.1b) can be organized into three groups: those that inhibit the flow of electrons, those that interfere with the flow of protons, and miscellaneous compounds.

Interference with the flow of electrons
(Diagram 3.1a)

(i) Rotenone, piericidin and Amytal. Ubiquinone (Q) is reduced to ubiquinol (QH_2), which shuttles between complexes I and III and, in so doing, transports electrons from complex I to complex III. Rotenone, piericidin and Amytal prevent the transfer of electrons from complex I to ubiquinone.

(ii) Malonate. Malonate, being structurally similar to succinate, is a competitive inhibitor of succinate dehydrogenase, which is a component of complex II.

(iii) Thenoyltrifluoroacetone. Ubiquinone can also shuttle electrons from complex II to complex III. This is inhibited by **thenoyltrifluoroacetone**, which prevents the transfer of electrons from complex II to ubiquinone.

(iv) Antimycin A and myxothiazol. Cytochrome c, which is loosely associated with the outer face of the inner membrane, shuttles electrons from complex III to complex IV. The transfer of electrons from complex III to cytochrome c is inhibited by antimycin A, and more potently by myxothiazol.

(v) Cyanide, carbon monoxide and azide. Electrons are transferred from complex IV (also known as cytochrome c oxidase) to molecular oxygen. This process is inhibited by cyanide, carbon monoxide and azide.

Interference with the flow of protons (H^+)
(Diagram 3.1b)

(i) Oligomycin and dicyclohexylcarbodiimide (DCCD). These compounds block the proton channel of the F_o segment of ATP synthetase. Consequently the flux of protons needed for ATP synthesis by the enzyme is prevented.

(ii) 2,4-dinitrophenol (DNP) and carbonylcyanide-*p*-trifluoromethoxy-phenylhydrazone (FCCP). Dinitrophenol (ditto FCCP) is a weak acid. Its base 2,4-dinitrophenate accepts H^+ producing the undissociated acid form, 2,4-dinitrophenol, which is lipophilic and diffuses across the inner mitochondrial membrane. This leakage of H^+ diverts the flux of H^+ from the ATP synthetase thus bypassing ATP synthesis. However, the flow of electrons is unrestricted by DNP and its effect is described as 'uncoupling ATP synthesis from electron transport'.

(iii) Uncoupling protein (UCP) that occurs in the inner mitochondrial membrane of brown adipose tissue and is involved in thermogenesis. Like DNP and FCCP, it lowers the electrochemical gradient by allowing leakage of protons so that energy is dissipated as heat instead of being used for ATP synthesis.

Some other compounds that affect the respiratory chain

(i) Tetramethyl-*p*-phenyldiamine (TMPD). TMPD is an artificial electron donor that can transfer electrons to cytochrome c. Since ascorbate can reduce TMPD, these compounds can be used experimentally to study the respiratory chain, Diagram 3.1a.

(ii) Bongkrekic acid and atractyloside. Bongkrekic acid (a toxic contaminant of bongkrek, which is a food prepared from coconuts) and atractyloside, both inhibit the ATP/ADP translocase preventing the export of ATP and the import of ADP. Whereas bongkrekic acid binds to the inner aspect of the adenine nucleotide carrier, atractyloside binds to its outer aspect.

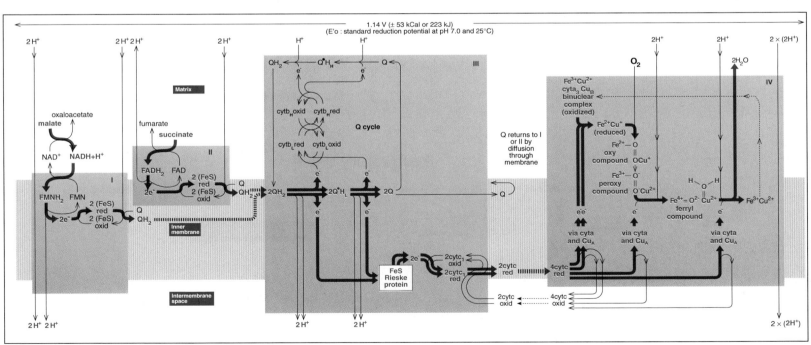

Diagram 3.2 This shows complexes I, II, III and IV in detail. **Complex I:** Protons and electrons from NADH are passed to FMN. The electrons pass to the iron/sulphur complex then to ubiqinone (Q), which also gains 2 H^+ and is reduced to ubiquinol (QH_2). **Complex II:** Electrons are passed from $FADH_2$ via the iron/sulphur complex to ubiquinone and are joined by protons to form ubiquinol. **Complex III:** Here ubiquinol delivers the protons which are extruded into the intermembrane space. Meanwhile, electrons are passed via the iron/sulphur Rieske protein and membrane-bound cytochrome c_1 before leaving the complex by reducing the cytosolic cytochrome c.

The 'Q cycle' is a device for regenerating ubiquinone from ubiquinone semiquinone $Q^\bullet H$ involving two cytochrome b's. **Complex IV:** Cytochrome c donates two electrons (indirectly via Cu_A and $haem_a$) to the oxidized binuclear complex $cyta_3Cu_B$. The resulting reduced complex binds O_2 to form the oxy species which rearranges to the peroxy form. Protonation and addition of a third electron, followed by oxygen–oxygen bond splitting produce the ferryl compound. A fourth electron and further protonation produce intermediates (not shown) which form water and regenerate the oxidized complex completing the cycle.

The oxidation of cytosolic NADH: the malate/aspartate shuttle and the glycerol phosphate shuttle

Oxidation of cytosolic NADH

The **glyceraldehyde 3-phosphate dehydrogenase** reaction occurs in the cytosol and forms NADH, which can be oxidized by the respiratory chain in the mitochondrion to produce ATP. However, molecules of NADH are unable to cross the inner membrane of the mitochondrion. This paradox is overcome by two mechanisms which enable 'reducing equivalents' to be transferred from the cytosol to the mitochondrion. They are the **malate/aspartate shuttle** and the **glycerol phosphate shuttle**.

The glycerol phosphate shuttle

This shuttle (below), which is particularly important in insects, uses the cytosolic NADH in the presence of **glycerol 3-phosphate dehydrogenase** to reduce **dihydroxyacetone phosphate** to form **glycerol 3-phosphate**. The latter diffuses into the intermembrane space of the mitochondrion. Here it is oxidized by the mitochondrial glycerol 3-phosphate dehydrogenase isoenzyme, which is associated with the outer surface of the inner membrane. The products of the reaction are dihydroxyacetone phosphate (which diffuses back into the cytosol) and $FADH_2$. This $FADH_2$ can be oxidized by the respiratory chain but, since it donates its electrons to ubiquinone (Q), there is enough energy to pump only six H^+. These can synthesize the equivalent of 1.5 molecules of ATP.

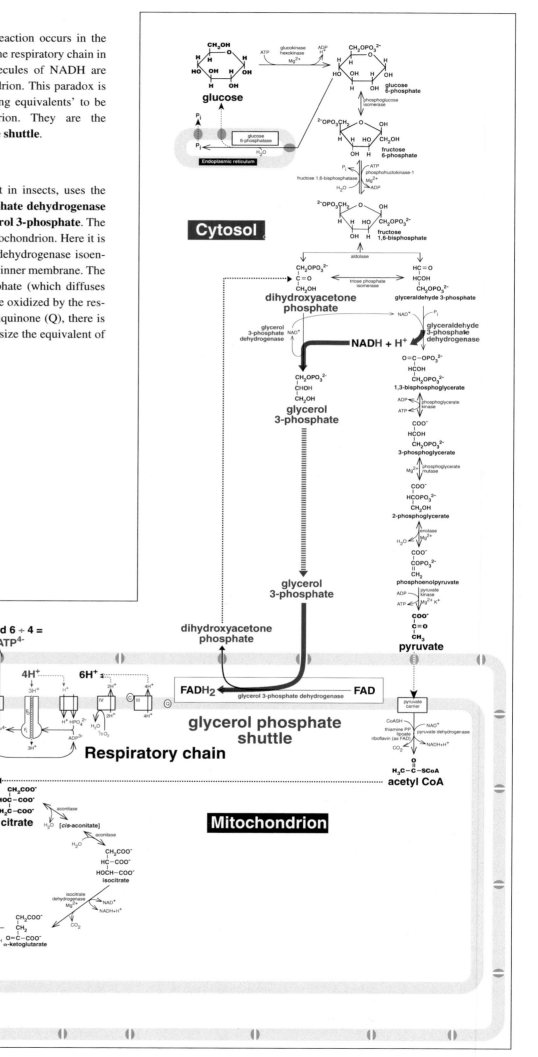

Chart 4.1 The glycerol phosphate shuttle.

The malate/aspartate shuttle

This shuttle (below) starts with cytosolic **oxaloacetate**. First, **cytosolic malate dehydrogenase** uses the NADH to reduce oxaloacetate to malate. The latter is transported into the mitochondrial matrix in exchange for α-ketoglutarate. Here it is oxidized by malate dehydrogenase back to oxaloacetate, and the NADH released is available for oxidative phosphorylation by the respiratory chain, producing ATP.

The oxaloacetate must now be returned to the cytosol. The problem is that it too is unable to cross the inner mitochondrial membrane. Accordingly, it is transformed to **aspartate** in a reaction catalysed by aspartate aminotransferase. Aspartate leaves the mitochondrion via the glutamate/aspartate carrier in exchange for the import of glutamate and a proton. Once in the cytosol, aspartate is transaminated by aspartate aminotransferase, and thus oxaloacetate is restored to the cytosol, thereby completing the cycle.

NB: Oxidation of each mitochondrial NADH in the respiratory chain provides energy to pump **10** H^+. However, since **1** H^+ is needed for the glutamate/aspartate carrier, a total of **9** H^+ are available to synthesize the equivalent of 2.25 molecules of ATP.

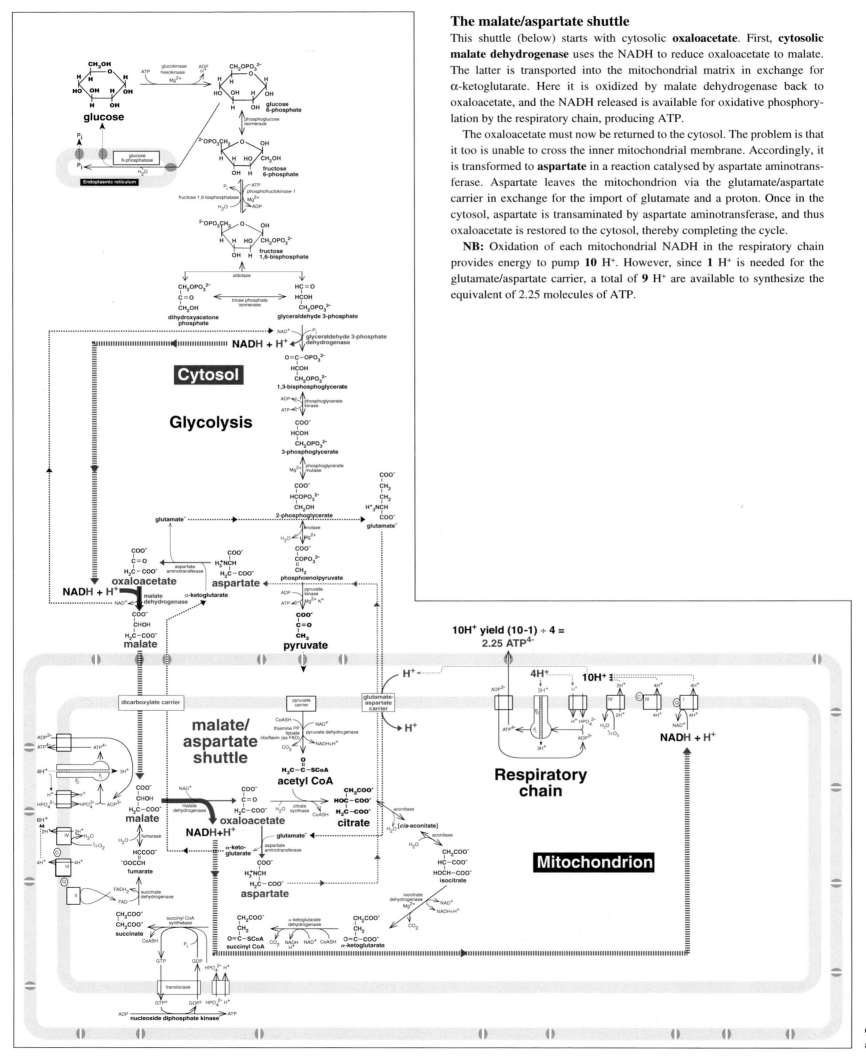

Chart 4.2 The malate/aspartate shuttle.

Metabolism of glucose to provide energy

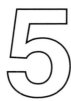

The glucose molecule, which is a rich store of chemical energy, burns vigorously in air to form carbon dioxide and water and, in the process, energy escapes as heat. This can be represented by the following equation:

$$C_6H_{12}O_6 + 6\,O_2 \longrightarrow 6\,CO_2 + 6\,H_2O + \text{energy as heat}$$

glucose   oxygen   carbon dioxide   water

Carbohydrate-containing foods such as starch are digested to glucose, which is then absorbed into the blood, and it is well known that 'glucose gives you energy'. Bearing in mind that the laws of thermodynamics apply to both animate and inanimate systems, we must now consider how living cells can release energy from a glucose molecule in a controlled way, so that the cell neither bursts into flames nor explodes in the process.

Once a glucose molecule has passed from the bloodstream into a cell, it is gradually transformed and dismantled in a controlled sequence of some two dozen biochemical steps, in a manner analogous to a production line in a factory. The several biochemical transformations are assisted by enzymes, some of which need cofactors derived from vitamins to function properly. Such a series of biochemical reactions is known as a metabolic pathway.

Chart 5.1: Glucose metabolism

The chart shows that, in order to conserve the energy from glucose as ATP, three metabolic pathways are involved. First, glucose is oxidized through the pathway known as **glycolysis**. The end product of glycolysis, two molecules of **pyruvate**, are then fed into **Krebs cycle**, where they are completely oxidized to form six molecules of carbon dioxide. In the process, the hydrogen carriers **NAD$^+$** and **FAD**, which are compounds derived from the vitamins niacin and riboflavin respectively, become reduced to **NADH** and **FADH$_2$** and carry hydrogen to the **respiratory chain**. Here, energy is conserved in **ATP** molecules, while the hydrogen is eventually used to reduce oxygen to water (see Chapter 3).

The energy released from ATP on hydrolysis can then be used for biological work such as muscle contraction, protein synthesis and conduction of nerve impulses.

Several vitamins provide cofactors for the enzymes involved in these metabolic pathways. For example, the pyruvate dehydrogenase reaction needs cofactors derived from niacin, thiamine, riboflavin, lipoic acid and pantothenic acid. A deficiency of any of these could cause malfunctioning of a metabolic pathway at the particular enzymic reaction(s) where the cofactor is involved.

The overall reaction for the oxidation of glucose by living cells is therefore:

$$C_6H_{12}O_6 + 6\,O_2 \longrightarrow 6\,CO_2 + 6\,H_2O + \text{energy as ATP}$$

glucose   oxygen   carbon dioxide   water

The importance of insulin in glucose transport

Insulin is a hormone secreted into the blood by the β cells of the pancreas in response to increased blood glucose concentrations such as might follow a carbohydrate meal. Because of the large mass of muscle and fat tissue in the human body, the ability of insulin to control the uptake and metabolism of glucose in these cells plays a major part in regulating the blood glucose concentration. In diabetes mellitus, where there is inadequate insulin action, glucose cannot enter muscle and fat cells and consequently the blood glucose concentration rises (hyperglycaemia). This situation has inspired the aphorism describing diabetes as 'starvation in the midst of plenty'.

If there is an inappropriate excess of insulin relative to the available glucose, then a low blood glucose concentration (hypoglycaemia) results. This might arise if a diabetic patient receives too much insulin in proportion to the carbohydrate supply – or in other words, fails to achieve the balance essential to diabetic control. A rare example of excessive insulin secretion occurs in patients with an insulin-secreting tumour (insulinoma) where the β cells are overactive. In both cases, the resulting hypoglycaemia is dangerous because the brain, which is largely dependent on glucose for fuel, is deprived of its energy supply, and coma may follow.

Insulin is a very important hormone. It has a controlling influence on the metabolism of fats and proteins as well as a direct involvement with glucose metabolism. Its many metabolic actions will be mentioned throughout this book.

Diagram 5.1 Insulin and the transport of glucose into muscle cells. As shown in Diagram 5.1, glucose is carried by the blood arterial system to the capillaries, which supply the various body tissues. Glucose penetrates the gaps in the capillary wall to form an aqueous fluid, called the interstitial fluid, which bathes the cells. In the case of erythrocytes, liver cells and brain cells, glucose is transported through the outer membrane into the cytosol via a family of insulin-independent facilitative glucose transporters known respectively as GLUT1, GLUT2 and GLUT3. However, in the case of muscle cells (see Diagram, which is not to scale) and fat cells, insulin-dependent glucose transporters are involved. Here, insulin is needed to recruit glucose transporters (of the GLUT4 type) from a latent intracellular location. Insulin causes a vesicle containing the glucose transporters to fuse with the sarcolemma, thereby stimulating glucose transport into the sarcoplasm, where it is oxidized and ATP is formed.

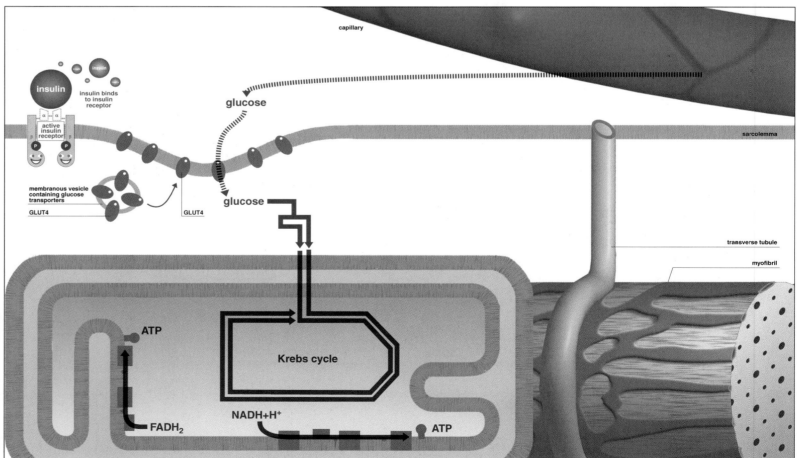

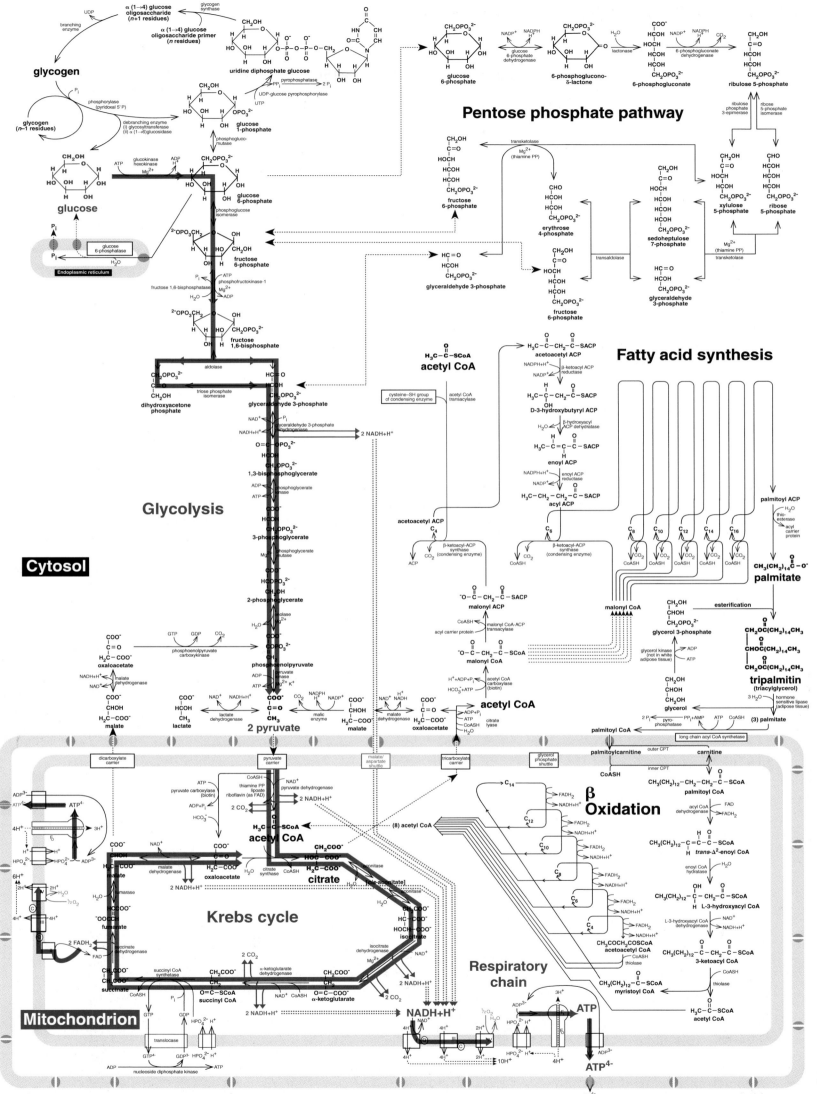

Chart 5.1 Metabolism of glucose to provide energy.

Metabolism of one molecule of glucose yields 31 (or should it be 38?) molecules of ATP

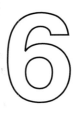

Warning! In what may appear to be a conspiracy to confuse students, the yield of ATP molecules from the oxidation of glucose, traditionally quoted as 38, is now cited as 31 in the new biochemistry textbooks. This is because experimental evidence for the P/O ratios for NADH and $FADH_2$ has, for more than 50 years, been interpreted as **whole number (i.e. integral)** values of **3** and **2** respectively. Recently, reinterpretation of the experimental evidence suggests that the P/O ratios are **non-integral** values of **2.5** for

NADH and **1.5** for $FADH_2$ (see Chapter 3). Using the traditional, integral values for P/O ratios, glucose oxidation produces 38 ATP. On the other hand, if non-integral P/O values are assumed, the yield from glucose is only 31 molecules of ATP.

Chart 6.1: Oxidation of glucose yields 38 ATP molecules assuming the traditional P/O ratios of 3 for NADH and 2 for $FADH_2$

On entering the cell glucose is phosphorylated to **glucose 6-phosphate**, a reaction which consumes one molecule of ATP. Glucose 6-phosphate then enters glycolysis and is converted through a series of hexose phosphates to **fructose 1,6-bisphosphate**, requiring yet another ATP molecule to be consumed. Thus, so far, instead of creating ATP, glycolysis has consumed two molecules of this source of biochemical energy. This initial investment of energy, however, is necessary to activate the substrates, and as we will see, is amply rewarded by a 19-fold (or 15.5-fold!?) net gain.

Fructose 1,6-bisphosphate is then split into two 3-carbon sugars, namely dihydroxyacetone phosphate and glyceraldehyde 3-phosphate. These two substances (triose phosphates) are biochemically interconvertible. Because two molecules of triose phosphate are formed, all subsequent reactions are doubled up and are represented in the chart by double lines.

Oxidation of glyceraldehyde 3-phosphate, and phosphorylation using inorganic phosphate, occur to form 1,3-bisphosphoglycerate. This complex oxidation reaction is catalysed by glyceraldehyde-3-phosphate dehydrogenase, and the NADH formed diffuses through the cytoplasm, exchanging its hydrogen through the impermeable inner membrane of the mitochondrion with assistance from one of the **shuttle systems** (see Chapter 4). In Chart 6.1 for example, the **malate/aspartate** shuttle has been used. The NADH formed in the mitochondrion then enters the respiratory chain, and three molecules of ATP are formed for each molecule of NADH oxidized.

Meanwhile, back in the glycolytic pathway, **phosphoglycerate kinase** causes 1,3-bisphosphoglycerate to react with ADP to form ATP and 3-phosphoglycerate. Similarly, two stages further down the pathway, pyruvate kinase causes phosphoenolpyruvate to react with ADP to form ATP and pyruvate. Pyruvate then passes into the mitochondrion and enters Krebs cycle, where $FADH_2$ and NADH are formed. $FADH_2$ is the prosthetic group attached to succinate dehydrogenase and donates its electrons via ubiquinone to complex III, and thence to complex IV. Accordingly, oxidative phosphorylation of $FADH_2$ produces only two ATP molecules compared with three from NADH (see Chapter 3). Also, it should be noted that in Krebs cycle, GTP is formed by the succinyl CoA synthetase reaction. GTP is energetically similar to ATP to which it is readily converted by nucleoside diphosphate kinase.

The net yield is 36 ATP molecules in insects

To add to the confusion, biochemistry textbooks may appear to contradict each other even when quoting the traditional yields of ATP from glucose

Chart 6.1 Oxidation of glucose yields **38** molecules of ATP.

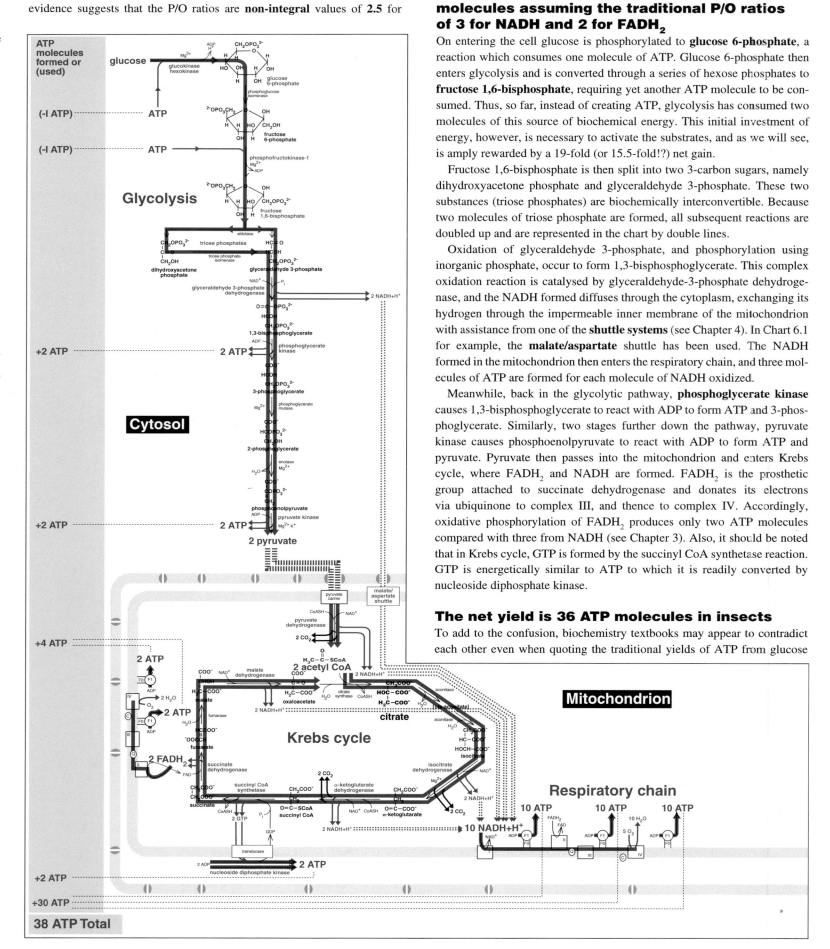

catabolism. Many books show the net energy yield for aerobic glucose metabolism to be **36** ATP molecules, and others give a value of **38** molecules as shown here.

The yield depends on which shuttle system (see Chapter 4) is used to transport cytosolic NADH into the mitochondrion. In the calculation shown in Chart 6.1 the malate/aspartate shuttle is used. However, if the glycerol phosphate shuttle is used, then 2 NADH molecules in the cytosol appear as 2 FADH$_2$ molecules inside the mitochondrion. The final yield of ATP is therefore 4 from the glycerol phosphate shuttle as opposed to 6 from the other shuttle. This accounts for the discrepancy referred to above. The glycerol phosphate shuttle is particularly active in insect flight muscle.

Chart 6.2: Oxidation of glucose yields 31 ATP molecules assuming the 'modern' P/O ratios of 2.5 for NADH and 1.5 for FADH$_2$

As shown in Chart 6.2 below, oxidation of the 10 NADH formed is coupled to the pumping of a total of 100 protons from the matrix into the intermembrane space. The return of 4 protons is needed to synthesize one ATP molecule and to translocate it to the cytosol (see Chapter 3). The total yield of ATP from 100 returning protons is therefore 25 molecules.

Similarly, oxidation of the 2 FADH$_2$ formed in Krebs cycle is coupled to the pumping of a total of 12 protons from the matrix into the intermembrane space. As before, the return of 4 protons is needed to synthesize one ATP molecule and to translocate it to the cytosol so the total yield from 12 returning protons is therefore 3 molecules of ATP.

Formation of GTP by substrate-level phosphorylation. In Krebs cycle, 2 molecules of GTP are formed within the mitochondrial matrix by the succinyl CoA synthetase reaction. These can be exported to the intermembrane space by a transport mechanism (see Chapter 4). This includes a **phosphate carrier** that requires the import of one proton for each GTP exported. In effect, this diverts 2 protons from ATP synthesis and is equivalent to the loss of 0.5 ATP molecules. Nevertheless, the 2 GTP molecules are metabolized to 2 ATP molecules by the **nucleoside diphosphate kinase** reaction and so there is a net gain of 1.5 molecules of ATP.

Malate/aspartate shuttle. If the 2 NADH reducing equivalents formed in the cytosol during glycolysis are translocated into the mitochondrion using the malate/aspartate shuttle, it must be remembered that the associated import of each glutamate anion needs the symport of a proton (see Chapter 4). Thus a total of 2 protons is diverted from ATP synthesis, which is a loss equivalent to 0.5 molecules of ATP. The total net gain from the oxidation of 2 molecules of NADH originating in the cytosol is therefore: $5 - 0.5 = 4.5$ molecules of ATP.

The net production of ATP molecules from the oxidation of one molecule of glucose when the malate/aspartate shuttle is used is 31.

Glycerol phosphate shuttle. The reducing power of NADH when translocated into the mitochondrion via the glycerol phosphate shuttle, is transformed into FADH$_2$ (see Chapter 4). Two molecules of FADH$_2$ yield a total of only 3 ATP molecules, which is $4.5 - 3 = 1.5$ less than the total via the malate/aspartate shuttle.

The net production of ATP molecules from the oxidation of one molecule of glucose, when the glycerol phosphate shuttle is used, is $31 - 1.5 = 29.5$.

Chart 6.2 (below). Oxidation of glucose yields **31** molecules of ATP.

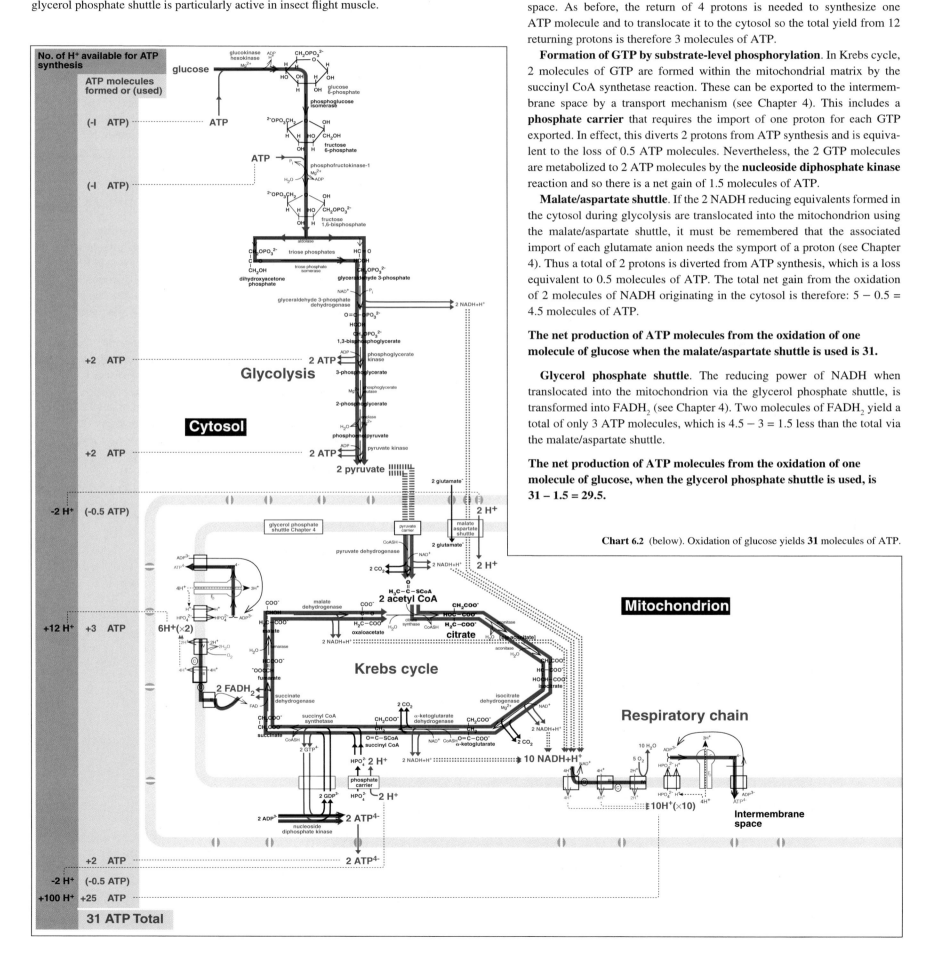

Metabolism of glucose to glycogen

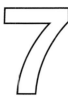

Glycogen is stored in the fed state

If we consume large quantities of carbohydrate-rich food in excess of our immediate requirements, then we might expect the concentration of glucose in the blood to rise higher and higher until it eventually assumed the consistency of syrup. If this happened, there would be serious osmotic implications, with water being drawn from the body's cells into the hypertonic blood, causing the former to become dehydrated.

Fortunately, apart from in the diabetic state, this sequence of events does not happen. We have evolved an elaborate control mechanism so that, when provided with a surplus of carbohydrate fuel, it is stored for less bountiful occasions either as **glycogen** or as fat. Glycogen is made from many glucose molecules joined together to form a compact, highly branched, spherical structure.

Chart 7.1: An overview of glycogen synthesis (glycogenesis)

The chart opposite shows how the metabolic fate of glucose can vary according to the energy status of the cell. As we saw in the previous chapter, if the cell needs energy and glucose is available, then the glucose will be oxidized by the glycolytic pathway, Krebs cycle and the respiratory chain, with the formation of ATP. If, however, the cell is supplied with surplus glucose, causing a high-energy state in the mitochondrion, then the capacity for metabolic flux through Krebs cycle is overwhelmed and certain metabolites accumulate. Some of these metabolites, such as **citrate**, and **ATP** from the respiratory chain, symbolize an energy surplus and act as messengers (allosteric inhibitors), which inhibit glycolysis. Thus in liver and muscle some of the excess glucose is channelled along the metabolic pathway to glycogen, a process known as **glycogenesis**.

Glycogen as a fuel reserve

The liver and muscles are the major depots for this important energy reserve. The average man who has been well fed on a diet rich in carbohydrate stores 70 g of glycogen in his liver and 200 g in his muscles. The liver glycogen reserves are sufficient only for an overnight fast at the longest. Accordingly the fat reserves must also be used, especially during long periods of fasting or strenuous exercise.

As we will see later, the brain cannot use fat directly as a fuel and is mainly dependent upon a steady supply of glucose via the blood. If the brain is denied glucose it ceases to function properly. The symptoms of a low plasma glucose level include a feeling of dizziness, faintness or lethargy. In hypoglycaemia, defined as a plasma glucose less than 2.5 mmol/l, these symptoms can progress to unconsciousness, coma and, unless glucose is provided rapidly, death.

We can now appreciate the great importance of the reserves of glucose stored as glycogen in the liver. We survive between meals because the liver is able to keep the blood glucose 'topped up' and can maintain a fasting blood concentration of 3.5–5.5 mmol/l, which satisfies the pernickety fuel requirements of the brain.

Glycogen is also an important energy source when confronted with a 'fight or flight' situation. This role will be discussed fully later (see Chapters 16–19) but, as we will see below, the structure of the glycogen molecule is beautifully adapted for the rapid mobilization of glucose in an emergency.

Diagram 7.1: Glycogen, a molecule that is well designed for its function

Glycogen is a complex hydrated polymer of glucose molecules which form a highly branched spherical structure. The very large molecular weight, which ranges over several million daltons, enables glucose to be stored without the osmotic complications associated with free glucose molecules. The size of the glycogen molecule varies with the prevailing nutritional status, being larger (up to 40 nm in diameter) in the fed state, and progressively shrinking to around 10 nm or less between meals.

The glucose chain is attached to the protein **glycogenin**. The glucose molecules are joined by $\alpha(1\rightarrow4)$glycosidic bonds, except at the branch points, which are $\alpha(1\rightarrow6)$glycosidic bonds. A branch occurs, on average, every 10 glucose units along the chain. This highly branched spherical structure creates a large number of exposed terminal glucose molecules, which are accessible to the enzymes involved in glycogen breakdown (glycogenolysis). This ensures an extremely rapid release of glucose units from glycogen in the 'fight or flight' emergency situation, which can sometimes be vital for survival.

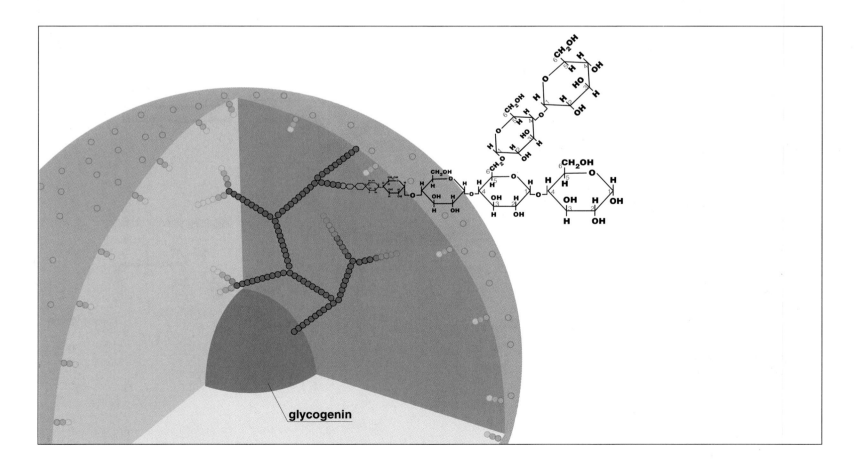

glycogenin

Diagram 7.1 Diagrammatic representation of a glycogen molecule.

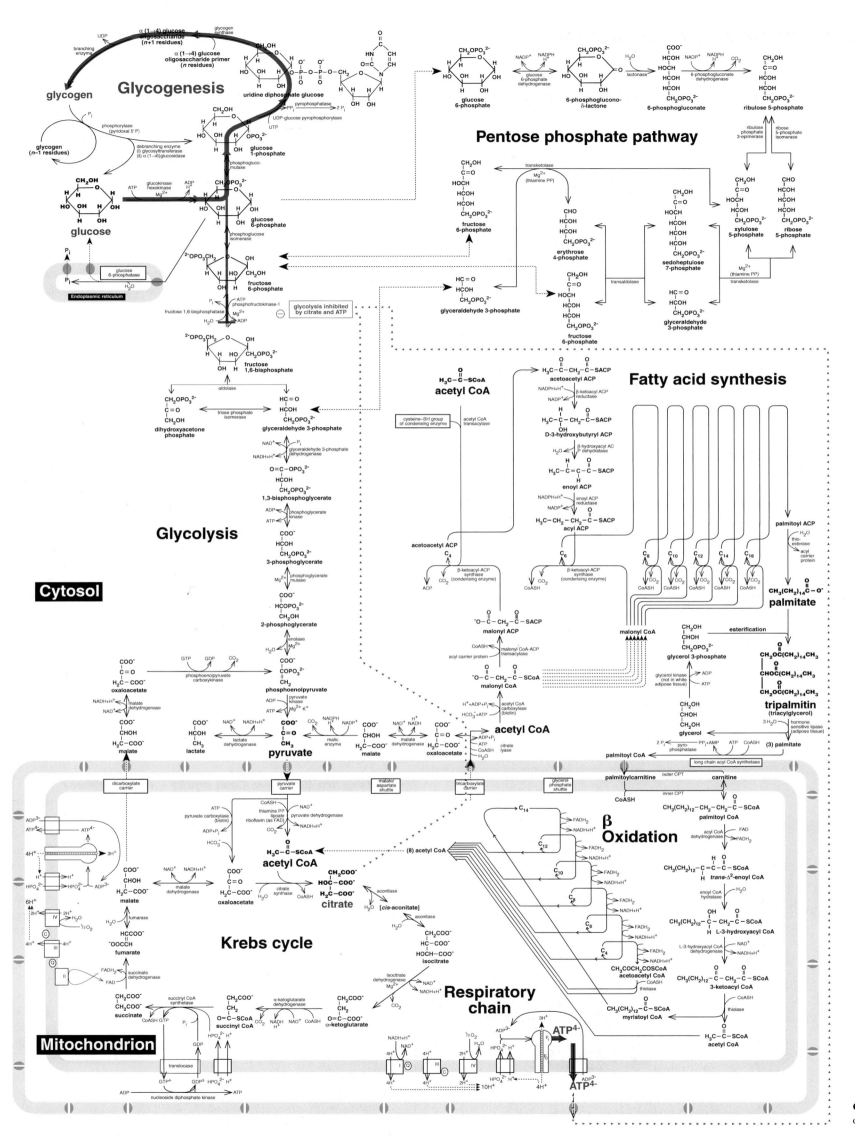

Chart 7.1 Metabolism of glucose to glycogen.

Anaerobic metabolism of glucose and glycogen to yield energy as ATP

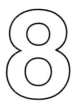

Anaerobic glycolysis

We have already seen how, in the presence of oxygen, glucose and glycogen are oxidized to carbon dioxide and water, with energy being conserved as ATP (see Chapter 6). However, glucose and glycogen can also be oxidized **anaerobically**: that is, without oxygen. This process is particularly important in exercising muscle. It enables muscle to generate ATP very rapidly and at a rate faster than would be permitted by the availability of oxygen from the air. In practice, this means that eventually we become 'out of breath' and then have to rest to repay the 'oxygen debt'.

Anaerobic glycolysis is also very important in the retina, kidney medulla and, paradoxically, in red blood cells in spite of the abundance of oxygen in the latter, see below.

Chart 8.1: Glucose is metabolized to lactate

Anaerobic oxidation proceeds as shown in the chart. **Glucose** and **glycogen** are metabolized by glycolysis to **pyruvate** and four ATP molecules are produced. However, NAD$^+$ is reduced to NADH by **glyceraldehyde 3-phosphate dehydrogenase**. Normally, in the presence of oxygen, this NADH equivalent (see Chapter 4) would enter the mitochondria and be oxidized to regenerate NAD$^+$. Since glycolysis needs a constant supply of NAD$^+$, the problem is how is NAD$^+$ regenerated without oxygen?

The enzyme **lactate dehydrogenase** provides the answer. This enzyme catalyses the reduction of pyruvate to **lactate**, and simultaneously NADH is oxidized to NAD$^+$. The regenerated NAD$^+$ is thus free to serve glyceraldehyde 3-phosphate dehydrogenase as a coenzyme. In this way, glycolysis continues but lactate accumulates. This represents the 'oxygen debt', which must be repaid, when oxygen is available, by oxidizing the accumulated lactate to pyruvate in the liver. The pyruvate formed is converted to glucose.

ATP yield by anaerobic metabolism

Anaerobic glycolysis from glucose

Molecules of ATP formed	4
Less 2 ATP to activate glycolysis	−2
Net ATP total	2

Anaerobic glycolysis from glycogen

Molecules of ATP formed	4
Less 1 ATP to initiate glycolysis	−1
Net ATP total	3

The above anaerobic pathways, which produce a net yield of two and three ATP molecules respectively, are very inefficient compared with the net yield from aerobic pathways, namely 31 molecules of ATP (see Chapter 6). Nevertheless, the ability to generate ATP rapidly in the absence of oxygen is vital to the survival of many species.

Physiological and clinical relevance
Anaerobic glycolysis for 'fuel-injection' performance

Adrenaline (epinephrine), as part of the 'fight or flight' response, stimulates the breakdown of glycogen and thus glycolysis. This pathway is especially important in fast-twitch (white) muscle, which is relatively deficient in oxidative metabolism due to a poor blood supply and few mitochondria. White muscle is found, for example, in the flight muscles of some game birds (e.g. grouse). It is well adapted for an explosive burst of energy, thus helping these animals to evade predators. Human skeletal muscle consists of both red and white fibres.

When oxygen becomes more plentiful again, the rate of glycolysis falls dramatically as more efficient oxidation involving Krebs cycle is activated. This adaptation is known as the '**Pasteur effect**' after Louis Pasteur, who first observed this phenomenon in yeast.

Hyperlactataemia and lactic acidosis

The blood concentration of lactate is normally around 1 mmol/l. Since the pK of lactic acid is 3.86, it is completely dissociated to form lactate anions and hydrogen ions at normal blood pH. If the concentration of lactate is increased up to 5 mmol/l, this is known as hyperlactataemia. If it exceeds 5 mmol/l, and the bicarbonate buffer system is overwhelmed, the condition is described as lactic acidosis and the blood pH may decrease from the normal range of 7.35–7.45 to around pH 7 or below. Lactic acidosis may result from increased lactate production due to tissue hypoxia. Alternatively, it may also result from decreased removal of lactate by the liver for gluconeogenesis due to disease or a reduced hepatic blood supply.

Lactic acidosis and disease

Lactic acidosis is often due to the generalized tissue hypoxia associated with shock or congestive cardiac failure. Here, two factors contribute to lactate accumulation. These are an inadequate oxygen supply to the tissue, causing increased anaerobic glycolysis with increased lactate production, and a decreased clearance of lactate from the blood.

A mild hyperlactataemia may also occur in thiamine deficiency. This is because **pyruvate dehydrogenase** needs **thiamine** for activity and, consequently, removal of pyruvate is obstructed. Since lactate dehydrogenase activity is high in cells, it maintains pyruvate and lactate at equilibrium, so that when pyruvate accumulates so also does lactate.

Diagram 8.1: The Cori cycle – muscle/liver

If our muscles need energy in an emergency or for a sprint racing event such as a 200 m race, then most of the ATP used will be derived from anaerobic breakdown of muscle glycogen by glycolysis. The diagram shows that lactate formed during this process diffuses from the muscle into the capillaries, and is transported to the liver, entering the lobules via the hepatic arterioles. Then, provided the liver cells are adequately oxygenated, the lactate is oxidized to pyruvate which may be reconverted to glucose by the process known as gluconeogenesis (see Chapter 23). The glucose so formed may be exported from the liver via the central vein and thus made available again to the muscle for energy purposes or for storage as glycogen. This is known as 'the Cori cycle'.

The Cori cycle – red blood cells/liver

Mature red blood cells do not contain mitochondria and are therefore exclusively dependent on anaerobic oxidation of glucose for their ATP supply. The lactate produced diffuses from the red cell into the plasma and thence to the liver, where it is oxidized to pyruvate and may then be reconverted to glucose (the Cori cycle). In laboratory medicine, fluoride is used as a preservative for blood glucose samples from diabetic patients because it inhibits the glycolytic enzyme **enolase**, which converts 2-phosphoglycerate to phosphoenolpyruvate.

Diagram 8.1 The Cori cycle.

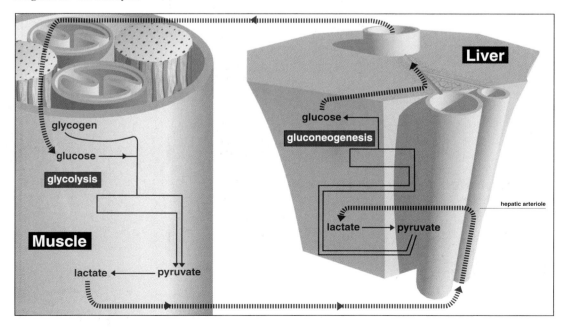

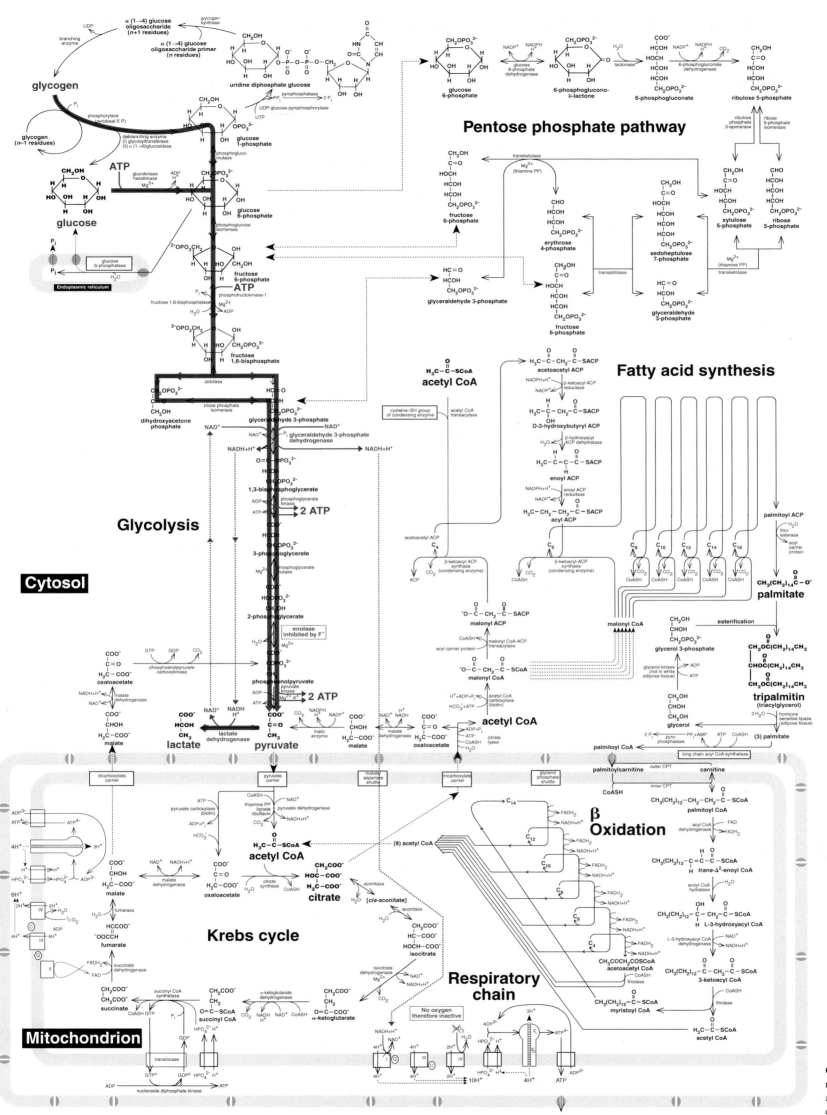

Chart 8.1 Anaerobic metabolism of glucose and glycogen to yield energy as ATP.

2,3-Bisphosphoglycerate (2,3-BPG) and the red blood cell

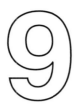

2,3-BPG helps to unload oxygen from haemoglobin

Haemoglobin, the oxygen-carrying protein found in red blood cells, has a high binding affinity for oxygen and can therefore transport oxygen to the tissues where it is needed. The problem then is that, on arrival at the tissues, haemoglobin must be persuaded to release its tightly bound cargo. It has been known since the early 1900s that the presence of H^+ ions in contracting muscle unloads oxygen from the haemoglobin. This is known as the 'Bohr effect'. However, it has been known only since 1967 that there is another factor, **2,3-BPG** (2,3-bisphosphoglycerate) – also known as 2,3-DPG (2,3-diphosphoglycerate) in medical circles – which is an allosteric effector that binds to deoxyhaemoglobin, thereby lowering its affinity for oxygen.

Whereas the response to H^+ ions is very rapid, 2,3-BPG operates over longer periods, allowing adaptations to gradual changes in oxygen availability.

Chart 9.1: The 2,3-BPG shunt in red blood cells (Rapoport–Luebering shunt)

The chart shows only glycolysis and the pentose phosphate pathway, since the other pathways shown in previous and subsequent chapters are not present in mature red blood cells.

The shunt consists of **bisphosphoglycerate mutase** and **2,3-bisphosphoglycerate phosphatase**. Bisphosphoglycerate mutase is stimulated by 3-phosphoglycerate causing increased production of 2,3-BPG. **NB:** When this shunt operates, ATP is not produced by the phosphoglycerate kinase reaction. This means that ATP is produced exclusively by the pyruvate kinase reaction, but there is no net gain of ATP from glycolysis under these circumstances.

Physiological significance of 2,3-BPG
Fetal haemoglobin has a low affinity for 2,3-BPG

Fetal haemoglobin is a tetramer of two α-chains and two γ-chains, unlike adult haemoglobin, which comprises two α- and two β-chains. Fetal haemoglobin has a lower affinity for 2,3-BPG than adult haemoglobin, and consequently it has a higher affinity for oxygen. This facilitates placental exchange of oxygen from the mother to the fetus.

2,3-BPG and adaptation to high altitude

Anyone accustomed to living at low altitude who has flown to a high-altitude location will be aware that even moderate exertion will cause breathlessness. Within a few days, adaptation occurs as the concentration of 2,3-BPG in red cells increases, enabling the tissues to obtain oxygen in spite of its relatively diminished availability in the thin mountain air. On returning to low altitude the concentration of 2,3-BPG, which has a half-life of 6 hours, returns rapidly to normal.

Importance of 2,3-BPG in medicine
Blood transfusions

Haematologists have long known that blood which has been stored prior to transfusion has an unusually high affinity for oxygen. This is because 2,3-BPG, which forms 65% of the organic phosphates of red cells, disappears on storing in acid-citrate–glucose medium, the concentration falling from about 5 mmol/l to 0.5 mmol/l in 10 days. Consequently, in theory, it would be expected that if a patient is given a large volume of stored blood, the red cells would be unable to unload their oxygen and so, in spite of the presence of oxygen, tissue hypoxia would result. However, in modern clinical practice this is prevented by using anticoagulants and additives (e.g. saline, adenine, glucose, mannitol), which minimize depletion of 2,3-BPG.

Deficiency of red-cell glycolytic enzymes

Patients with inherited diseases due to deficiencies of red-cell glycolytic enzymes are unable to transport oxygen normally. However, the nature of the effect on 2,3-BPG concentrations depends on whether the deficiency is proximal or distal to the 2,3-BPG shunt. In patients with proximal deficiencies, for example **hexokinase**, **phosphoglucose isomerase**, **phosphofructokinase** and **aldolase** deficiencies, there is a reduced flow of metabolites through glycolysis, and consequently the 2,3-BPG concentration falls. There is therefore an associated tendency towards tissue hypoxia, since the haemoglobin maintains its high affinity for oxygen. In enzymopathies distal to the shunt, such as **pyruvate kinase** deficiency, the opposite situation prevails. Here, the glycolytic intermediates accumulate and, as a result, 2,3-BPG reaches about twice its normal concentration. This means that in this condition haemoglobin has a relatively low affinity for, and ability to transport, oxygen.

Finally, patients have been reported with deficiency of the shunt enzymes, **BPG mutase** and **2,3-BPG phosphatase**, suggesting that both activities reside in the same protein. As would be expected, concentrations of 2,3-BPG are severely decreased in these patients, who have an increase in red-cell mass to compensate for the diminished supply of oxygen to the tissues.

Hypophosphataemia during therapy for diabetic ketoacidosis

Hypophosphataemia may result from intravenous infusion of glucose post-operatively, or may occur after insulin treatment for diabetic ketoacidosis. This is because of the acute demand for phosphate by the tissues to form the phosphorylated intermediates of metabolism. Unfortunately, the fall in plasma phosphate causes low concentrations of phosphate in red cells. This results in decreased 2,3-BPG levels, which in turn causes tissue hypoxia.

It has been suggested that, during glucose infusion and during treatment for diabetic ketoacidosis, phosphate replacement might minimize tissue hypoxia and so assist recovery. However, clinical studies have shown that, whereas phosphate therapy might accelerate the regeneration of 2,3-BPG in red cells, there were no demonstrable clinical benefits to the patients.

Common causes of increased red-cell 2,3-BPG concentrations

The concentration of 2,3-BPG is increased in smokers, which compensates for a diminished oxygen supply because of their chronic exposure to carbon monoxide. Also, a compensatory increase in 2,3-BPG is commonly found in patients with chronic anaemia.

Myoglobin

Myoglobin is very similar to the β-chain of haemoglobin and it also has a high affinity for oxygen. Although 2,3-BPG has no direct effect on myoglobin, this important protein and its role in oxygen transport must not be overlooked. It provides a reserve supply of oxygen and, as such, is particularly abundant in the skeletal muscle of aquatic mammals such as whales and seals, enabling them to remain submerged for several minutes.

Diagram 9.1: Transport of oxygen from the red blood cell to the mitochondrion for use in oxidative phosphorylation

Diagram 9.1 shows the route by which oxygen is transported from haemoglobin to the mitochondrion. First, oxygen is dissociated from haemoglobin in red cells and diffuses through the capillary wall into the extracellular fluid, and on into the muscle cell. Here, oxygen is bound to myoglobin until required by complex IV of the respiratory chain for oxidative phosphorylation.

Reference

Fisher J.N. & Kitabchi A.E. (1983) A randomised study of phosphate therapy in the treatment of diabetic ketoacidosis. *J Clin Endocrinol Metab*, **57**, 177–80.

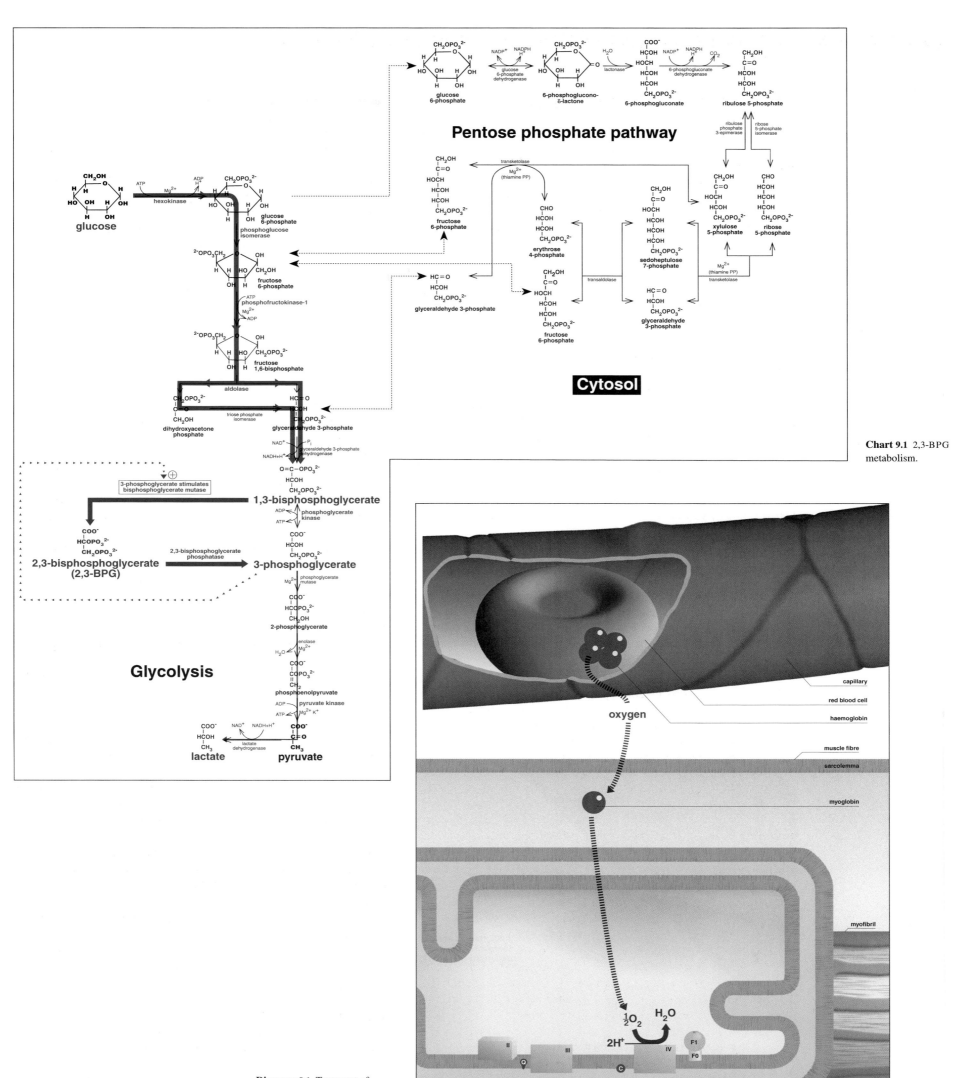

Chart 9.1 2,3-BPG metabolism.

Diagram 9.1 Transport of oxygen from the red blood cell to the mitochondrion for use in oxidative phosphorylation.

Metabolism of glucose to fat (triacylglycerol)

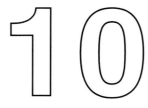

The importance of fat

The statement 'if you eat too much food, you will become fat' is unlikely to surprise any reader of this book. We know from experience that a surplus of fat in our diet will increase the fat in our body. Furthermore, it is general knowledge that an excess of carbohydrate will be stored as fat. However, a surprising number of people enjoy life under the delusion that they can eat large amounts of protein without the hazard of becoming obese. Sadly, this misconception will be shattered by reality in Chapter 39. Let us turn to the physiological advantages of body fat. Primitive man, like many other carnivorous mammals that hunted for food, was an intermittent feeder. In the days before refrigeration he was unable to store joints from his woolly mammoth in the deep-freeze, to be divided subsequently into a gastronomical routine of breakfast, lunch, dinner and supper. Instead, when food was available the hunters and their families ate all they could, with any surplus to immediate energy requirements being stored in the body, to a certain extent as glycogen but mainly as fat. This fat can provide an energy store for sustenance over periods of starvation lasting several days or even weeks.

Fat provides a very compact store for energy, largely because of its highly reduced and anhydrous nature. In fact, 1 g of fat yields 9 kcal (37 kJ). This compares well with 1 g of carbohydrate, 3.75 kcal (16 kJ), or 1 g of protein, 4 kcal (17 kJ).

Liver cells and fat cells (adipocytes) are both major producers of fat. In addition, with the onset of lactation at the end of pregnancy, the mammary gland develops almost overnight the ability to synthesize prodigious amounts of fat for secretion in the milk.

Chart 10.1: The flow of metabolites when glucose is converted to triacylglycerol

The chart shows the metabolic pathways involved when a surplus of carbohydrate is taken in the diet. We have seen how the liver is able to conserve useful, but limited, supplies of energy as glycogen (see Chapter 7). Once these glycogen reserves are full, any additional carbohydrate will be converted to fat as follows: glucose enters the pentose phosphate pathway, the metabolites of which form a temporary diversion from the glycolytic pathway. The metabolites eventually rejoin the main glycolytic route, pass into the mitochondrion and enter Krebs cycle. However, in the fed state the mitochondrial pathways will be working to capacity and generating large amounts of ATP and NADH. Under these circumstances, a control mechanism (see Chapter 24) diverts citrate from Krebs cycle into the cytosol for fatty acid synthesis (see Chapter 11). Although Chart 10.1 shows the formation of **palmitate**, stearate is also formed by this pathway. Both can be esterified and incorporated into **triacylglycerols**. **NB:** The vitamin **biotin** is an essential cofactor for the regulatory enzyme **acetyl CoA carboxylase** in the pathway for fatty acid synthesis.

Diagram 10.1: Insulin and fat synthesis

Adipocytes are the specialized cells of adipose tissue where triacylglycerols are synthesized and stored. They contain the usual cellular organelles but, because the cell interior is almost completely occupied by a large, spherical fat droplet, the cytosol and organelles are displaced to the periphery. Adipose tissue is widely distributed, being found beneath the skin and especially around the intestines, kidneys and other visceral organs.

Blood capillaries in adipose tissue bring supplies of glucose for fatty acid synthesis. The diagram shows the relationship between adipocytes and a capillary, but is not to scale: in reality, the adipocytes would be much larger. The glucose passes through the capillary wall into the extracellular fluid. After feeding, insulin is released from the pancreas and causes a 30-fold increased rate of transport of glucose into the adipocyte. Insulin causes the translocation of a latent pool of GLUT4 glucose transporters from within the adipocyte cytosol to the plasma membrane. These facilitate the transport of glucose into the cytosol, where it is metabolized to triacylglycerols, which are stored as a spherical droplet as described earlier.

Not all the body's triacylglycerol is made by the adipose tissue. Triacylglycerol is usually available in food and is absorbed from the gut as protein-phospholipid-coated packages known as chylomicrons, whose role is to transport the triacylglycerols from the intestines to the adipocytes for storage. Alternatively, the **liver** makes triacylglycerols from glucose for export in a similar package known as a VLDL (very low-density lipoprotein). Likewise, these VLDLs transport triacylglycerol to adipose tissue for storage.

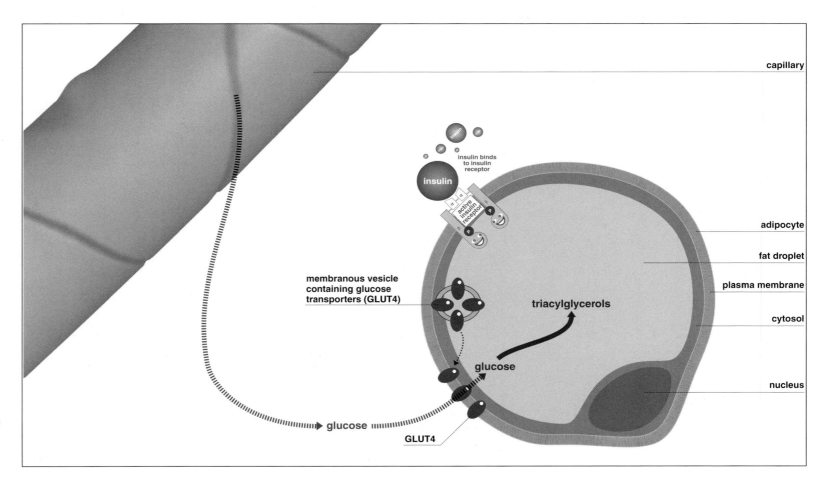

Diagram 10.1 Insulin stimulates the transport of glucose into adipocytes for triacylglycerol synthesis.

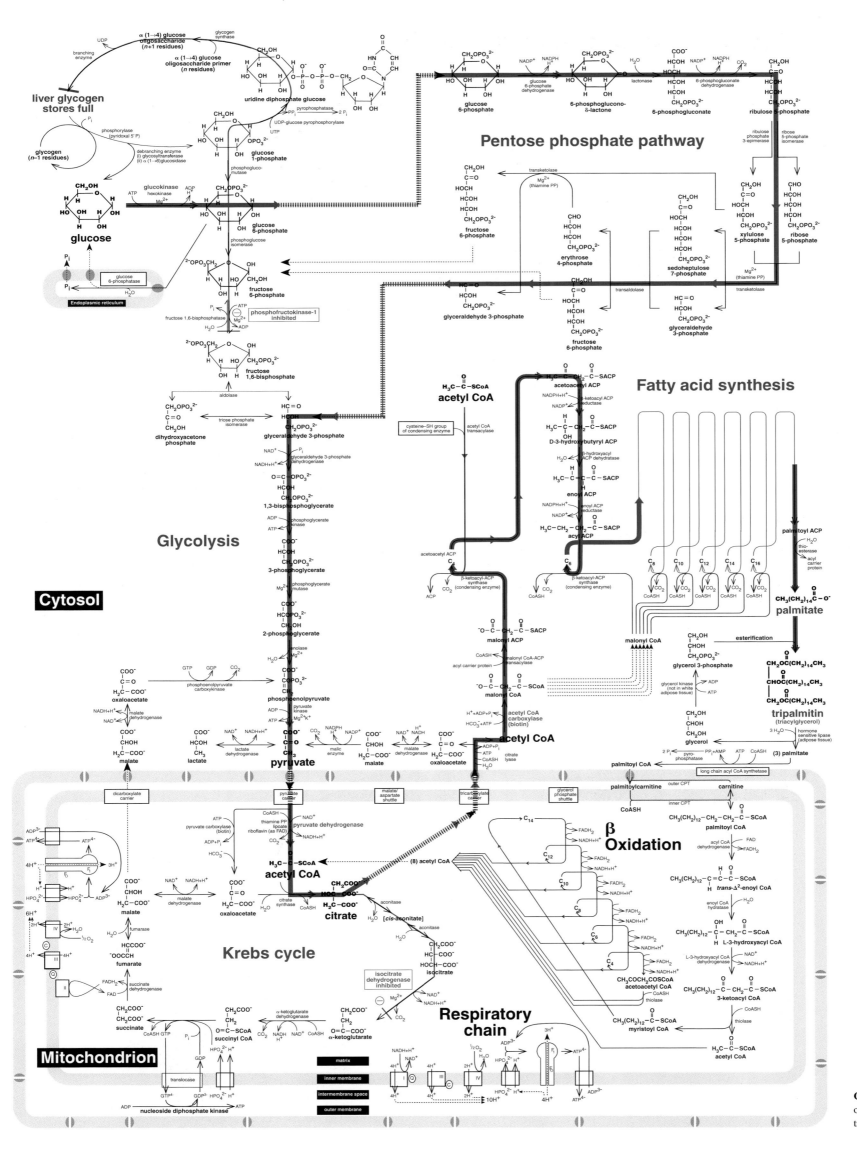

Chart 10.1 Metabolism of glucose to triacylglycerol.

Metabolism of glucose to fatty acids and triacylglycerol

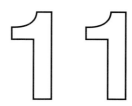

A brief description of how glucose is converted to fat appeared in Chapter 10. It is now time to look at triacylglycerol biosynthesis in more detail.

The liver, adipose tissue and lactating mammary gland are the principal tissues involved in lipogenesis (triacylglycerol synthesis). Liver and adipose tissue make triacylglycerol from glucose under conditions of abundant carbohydrate intake; in other words, when the body has more than enough food to satisfy its immediate needs for energy.

Chart 11.1: Synthesis of triacylglycerols from glucose
The importance of citrate in activating fatty acid synthesis

The mitochondrion in the high-energy state has increased amounts of ATP and NADH. These metabolites, both symbols of cellular affluence, reduce the rate of flow of metabolites through Krebs cycle by inhibiting **isocitrate dehydrogenase**. Consequently, the metabolites isocitrate and **citrate** accumulate, and their concentration within the mitochondrion increases. As the concentration of citrate rises, it diffuses via the **tricarboxylate carrier** from the mitochondrion into the cytosol, where citrate serves three functions:

1 Citrate and ATP are allosteric regulators that reduce the metabolic flux through glycolysis by inhibiting **phosphofructokinase-1**, thereby redirecting metabolites into the pentose phosphate pathway. This pathway produces NADPH, which is an essential coenzyme for fatty acid synthesis.
2 Citrate in the cytosol is split by **citrate lyase** (the citrate cleavage enzyme) to form **oxaloacetate** and **acetyl CoA**. The latter is the precursor for fatty acid synthesis.
3 Citrate activates **acetyl CoA carboxylase**, which is a regulatory enzyme controlling fatty acid synthesis.

In these three ways, citrate has organized the metabolic pathways of the liver or fat cell so that lipogenesis may proceed.

The pentose phosphate pathway generates NADPH for fatty acid synthesis

To reiterate, once the immediate energy demands of the animal have been satisfied, surplus glucose will be stored in the liver as glycogen. When the glycogen stores are full, any surplus glucose molecules will find the glycolytic pathway restricted at the level of phosphofructokinase. Under these circumstances, metabolic flux via the **pentose phosphate pathway** is stimulated. This is a complex pathway generating **glyceraldehyde 3-phosphate**, which then re-enters glycolysis, thus bypassing the restriction at phosphofructokinase-1. Because of this bypass, the pathway is sometimes referred to as the 'hexose monophosphate shunt' pathway.

One very important feature of the pentose phosphate pathway is that it produces NADPH from NADP$^+$. NADPH is a hydrogen carrier derived from the vitamin niacin, and as such is a phosphorylated form of NAD$^+$, the important functional difference being that, whereas NADH is used for ATP production, NADPH is used for fatty acid synthesis and other biosynthetic reactions.

Fatty acid synthesis and esterification

Starting from glucose, the chart shows the metabolic flux via the pentose phosphate pathway and glycolysis to mitochondrial acetyl CoA, and hence via citrate to acetyl CoA in the cytosol. Fatty acid synthesis is catalysed by the fatty acid synthase complex, which requires malonyl CoA. The latter combines with the **acyl carrier protein** (**ACP**) to form **malonyl ACP**. Fatty acid synthesis proceeds via the cyclical series of of reactions as shown in the chart to form **palmitate** (and also stearate, which is not shown). However, fat is stored not as fatty acids but as **triacylglycerols** (triglycerides). These are made by a series of esterification reactions that combine three fatty acid molecules with **glycerol 3-phosphate** (see Chapter 25).

Diagram 11.1: Activation of acetyl CoA carboxylase by citrate *in vitro*

Experiments *in vitro* have shown that acetyl CoA carboxylase exists as units (or protomers), which are enzymically inactive. However, citrate causes these protomers to polymerize and form enzymically active filaments that promote fatty acid synthesis. Conversely, the product of the reaction, namely fatty acyl CoA (palmitoyl CoA), causes depolymerization of the filaments. Kinetic studies have shown that, whereas polymerization is very rapid, taking only a few seconds, depolymerization is much slower, with a half-life of approximately 10 minutes. The length of a polymer varies, but on average consists of 20 units, and it has been calculated that a single liver cell contains 50 000 such filaments.

Each of the units contains biotin and is a dimer of two identical polypeptide subunits. The activity is also regulated by hormonally mediated phosphorylation/dephosphorylation reactions (see Chapter 25).

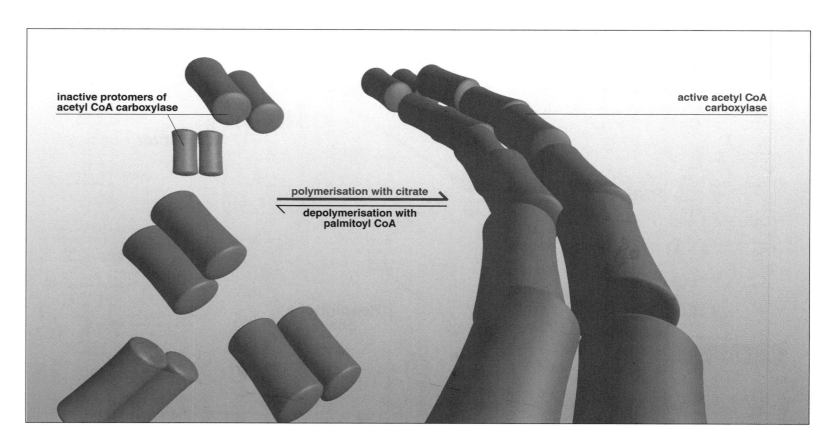

inactive protomers of acetyl CoA carboxylase

active acetyl CoA carboxylase

polymerisation with citrate

depolymerisation with palmitoyl CoA

Diagram 11.1 Activation of acetyl CoA carboxylase by citrate.

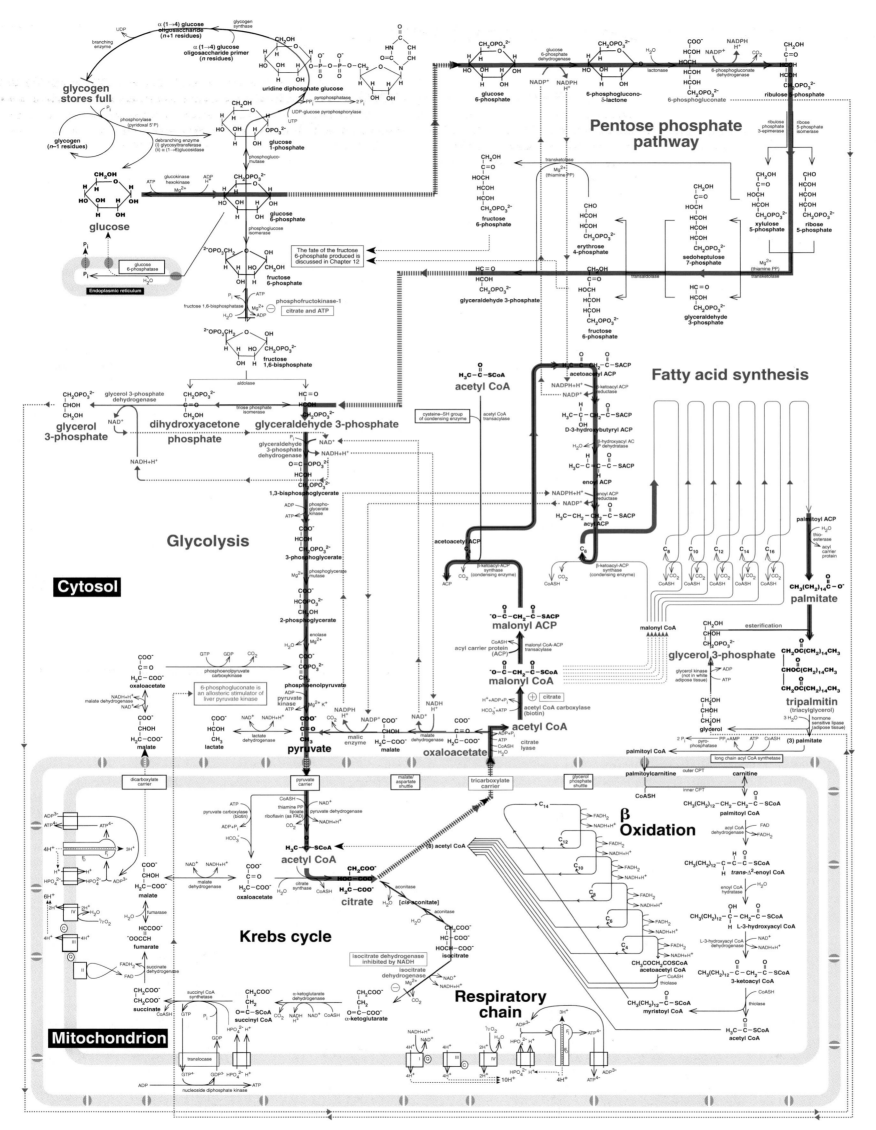

Chart 11.1 Metabolism of glucose to fatty acids and triacylglycerol.

The pentose phosphate pathway: the production of NADPH and reduced glutathione

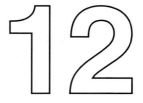

The pentose phosphate pathway

In mammals, the pentose phosphate pathway (also known as the hexose monophosphate shunt) is very active in liver, adipose tissue, lactating mammary gland, adrenal cortex and red blood cells. In these tissues it provides 'reducing power' in the form of NADPH. This NADPH is used for the biosynthesis of fatty acids, cholesterol and the production of reduced glutathione. The pathway is used by plants in the photosynthetic dark reaction.

Another important function is to produce ribose 5-phosphate for biosynthesis of purines and pyrimidines, nucleotides and nucleic acids. However, as described later, only the 'reversible, non-oxidative phase' of the pathway, which is ubiquitous, is needed for this process.

Chart 12.1: The pentose phosphate pathway

The pathway can be considered in two phases: the **irreversible oxidative phase** comprising the reactions catalysed by glucose 6-phosphate dehydrogenase, lactonase and 6-phosphogluconate dehydrogenase; and the **reversible, non-oxidative phase** involving the rest of the pathway.

Irreversible, oxidative phase of the pentose phosphate pathway

The stoichiometry of the pentose phosphate pathway can be studied by following the metabolic fate of three molecules of glucose. In the fed state, glucose is phosphorylated to **glucose 6-phosphate**. Remember that phosphofructokinase-1 (PFK-1) is inhibited by the abundance of ATP and citrate in the well-fed, high-energy state. Accordingly, glucose 6-phosphate enters the pentose phosphate pathway, where it is oxidized by **glucose 6-phosphate dehydrogenase** (G6-PDH) and NADPH is formed. Also produced is 6-phosphoglucono-δ-lactone, which is rapidly and irreversibly hydrolysed by **lactonase**. Next, **6-phosphogluconate dehydrogenase** irreversibly produces **ribulose 5-phosphate**, another molecule of NADPH is formed and CO_2 is evolved. Henceforth, the flux of metabolites is committed to the next 'reversible' phase of the pathway.

Reversible, non-oxidative phase of the pentose phosphate pathway

These reactions convert three molecules of **ribulose 5-phosphate** to two molecules of fructose 6-phosphate and one molecule of glyceraldehyde 3-phosphate. **NB:** Ribose 5-phosphate is a precursor of nucleotide synthesis.

The fate of fructose 6-phosphate

In red blood cells, for example (Chart 12.1), fructose 6-phosphate is converted to glucose 6-phosphate by the equilibrium reaction catalysed by **phosphoglucose isomerase** for re-entry into the pentose phosphate pathway. This cycle is especially important in cells prone to oxidative damage, for example, red blood cells, where the NADPH produced is used to synthesize **reduced glutathione**.

Alternatively, in the fed state in liver (Chart 12.2) and adipose tissue where lipogenesis prevails, fructose 6-phosphate is directed via glycolysis to pyruvate and then onwards for fatty acid synthesis (see Chapter 21). However, the inhibition of PFK-1 by citrate and ATP must be overcome (see Chapter 21).

Regulation of the pentose phosphate pathway

The flow of metabolites through the pathway is regulated at the glucose 6-phosphate dehydrogenase reaction and the 6-phosphogluconate dehydrogenase reaction by the availability of NADP+. Therefore, in red blood cells for example, the flow is linked to the availability of NADP+ provided by **glutathione reductase**; the latter is needed to produce **reduced glutathione**, which protects the cells from oxidative damage. In liver it is regulated by the availability of NADP+ supplied by fatty acid synthesis (see Chapter 21).

Glutathione: role as an antioxidant, in xenobiotic metabolism and in amino acid transport

Glutathione is a tripeptide that is formed from **glutamate**, **cysteine** and **glycine** as shown in Diagram 12.1. Glutathione protects cells against oxidative damage by removing hydrogen peroxide as shown in Chart 12.1. Glutathione is very abundant in liver (up to 10 mmol/l), where it has many functions. In particular it conjugates with fat-soluble toxins and drug metabolites to form water-soluble products for excretion. Another role is transporting amino acids across the plasma membrane into the cytosol by the 'γ-glutamyl cycle' (Diagram 12.1). Glutathione reacts with the amino acid to form the dipeptides 'γ-glutamyl-amino acid' and γ-cysteinylglycine in a reaction catalysed by **γ-glutamyltranspeptidase** (γ-GT). **γ-Glutamylcyclotransferase** then liberates the amino acid into the cytosol. **NB:** γ-GT is located on the outer surface of the plasma membrane and after consuming alcohol it is dislodged and appears in the plasma. Accordingly, it is a sensitive test for alcohol abuse.

Glucose 6-phosphate dehydrogenase deficiency

The most common inborn error of metabolism is glucose 6-phosphate dehydrogenase (G 6-PDH) deficiency which results in reduced production of NADPH by the pentose phosphate pathway. In affected individuals under normal circumstances, NADPH is produced in sufficient amounts to form reduced glutathione which prevents oxidative damage to red blood cells. Consequently, those people deficient in G 6-PDH are often unaware of their condition until severe oxidative stress is provoked by taking a drug such as primaquine which precipitates acute haemolysis and can damage up to 50% of the red blood cells. Other drugs causing acute anaemia in G 6-PDH deficiency include: sulphonamides, trinitrotoluene, methylene blue and nalidixic acid. The increased demand for NADPH when metabolizing such drugs renders the patient unable to maintain glutathione in its reduced state, hence the catastrophic oxidative damage to the red blood cells.

Favism

Some individuals with G 6-PDH deficiency suffer a haemolytic crisis after eating fava beans – also known as broad beans – (*Vicia fava*) which are a staple food in the Mediterranean region. This condition is known as favism. Surprisingly, sufferers from favism do not necessarily experience drug-induced haemolysis. There is no simple explanation for this apparent discrepancy.

Diagram 12.1 The γ-glutamyl cycle. This cycle forms glutathione from glutamate, cysteine and glycine. Extracellular amino acids combine with glutathione and enter the cell in the presence of the transmembrane enzyme, γ-glutamyl transpeptidase.

5-oxoprolinuria (pyroglutamic aciduria). Although usually associated with γ-glutamyl cycle defects, 5-oxoprolinuria also occurs in patients with other inborn errors e.g. urea cycle defects and organic acidurias.
This is probably because of reduced ATP availability in these conditions since ATP is needed by 5-oxoprolinase for 5-oxoproline degradation. 5-oxoprolinuria also occurs in hawkinsinuria secondary to glutathione depletion, see Chapter 41.

Chart 12.1 Pentose phosphate pathway in red blood cells. Red blood cells, which contain oxygen in high concentrations, are vulnerable to oxidative damage caused by peroxides. This is prevented by glutathione peroxidase, which needs reduced glutathione (GSH). GSH is regenerated from oxidized glutathione (GSSG) and NADPH formed in the pentose phosphate pathway.

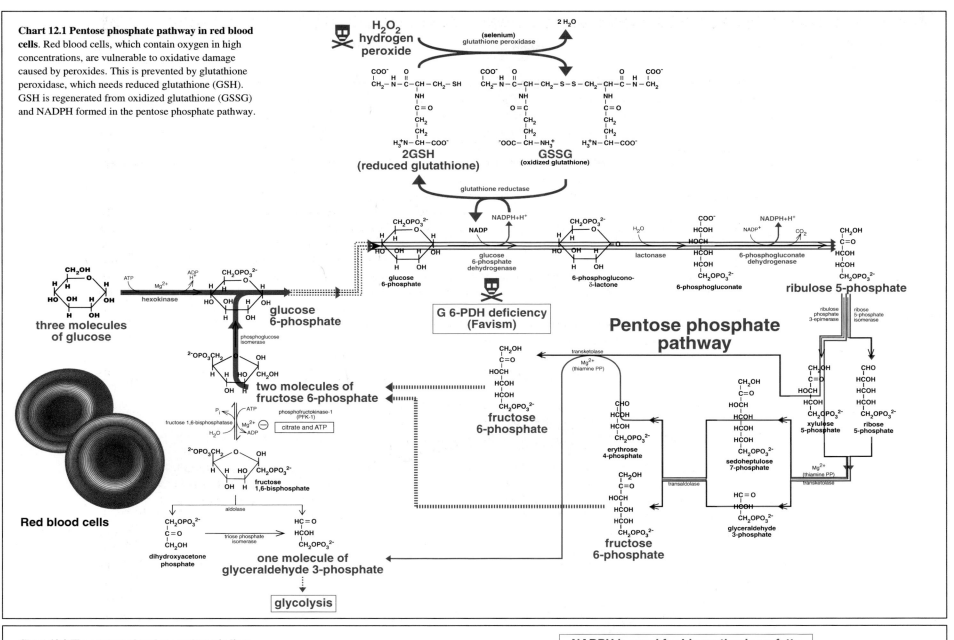

Chart 12.2 The pentose phosphate pathway in liver. The pathway produces NADPH, which is used for biosynthetic reactions. The fructose 6-phosphate formed is directed via glycolysis for fatty acid synthesis.

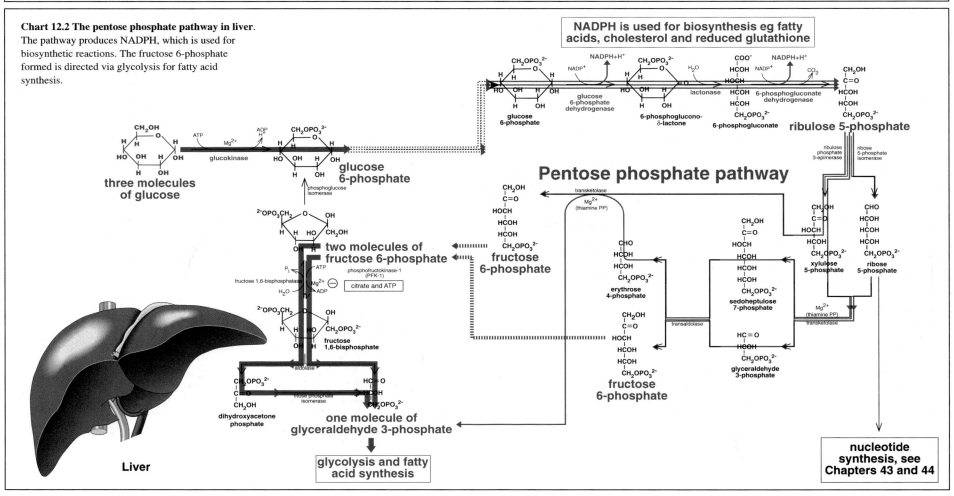

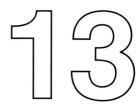

The pyruvate/malate cycle

The pyruvate/malate cycle has two main functions associated with lipogenesis: it transports acetyl CoA units from the mitochondrion into the cytosol, and it generates NADPH in the reaction catalysed by the **malic enzyme**.

Chart 13.1: The pyruvate/malate cycle

Fatty acid synthesis occurs in the cytosol. However, the carbon source, namely acetyl CoA, is produced by pyruvate dehydrogenase in the mitochondrion. Transport of acetyl CoA from the mitochondrion into the cytosol involves the **pyruvate/malate cycle**.

The principal stages are:

1 One molecule of pyruvate is carboxylated by **pyruvate carboxylase** to form **oxaloacetate**.

2 A second pyruvate molecule forms **acetyl CoA** by the **pyruvate dehydrogenase** reaction.

3 The acetyl CoA and oxaloacetate so formed condense to form citrate, which is transported to the cytosol for cleavage by **citrate lyase** to oxaloacetate and **acetyl CoA** for lipogenesis. Oxaloacetate is reduced by

Chart 13.2 Lactate as a substrate for fatty acid synthesis.

cytosolic malate dehydrogenase and **malate** is formed. Malate is oxidatively decarboxylated by the **malic enzyme** (malate dehydrogenase, decarboxylating) with the formation of NADPH, CO_2 and pyruvate, thus completing the cycle.

The relative contributions of the pentose phosphate pathway and the pyruvate/malate cycle to the provision of NADPH for fatty acid synthesis

For each acetyl unit added to the acyl ACP chain during the process of fatty acid synthesis, two molecules of NADPH are needed (see Chapter 11).

Experimental evidence suggests that if glucose is used for fatty acid synthesis, the pentose phosphate pathway supplies 60% of the NADPH needed with 40% produced by the pyruvate/malate cycle.

Fatty acid synthesis is also possible from other precursors, for example, amino acids (see Chapter 39) or lactate (see Chart 13.2). For instance, if lactate is used for fatty acid synthesis, only 25% of the NADPH needed is provided by the pyruvate/malate cycle.

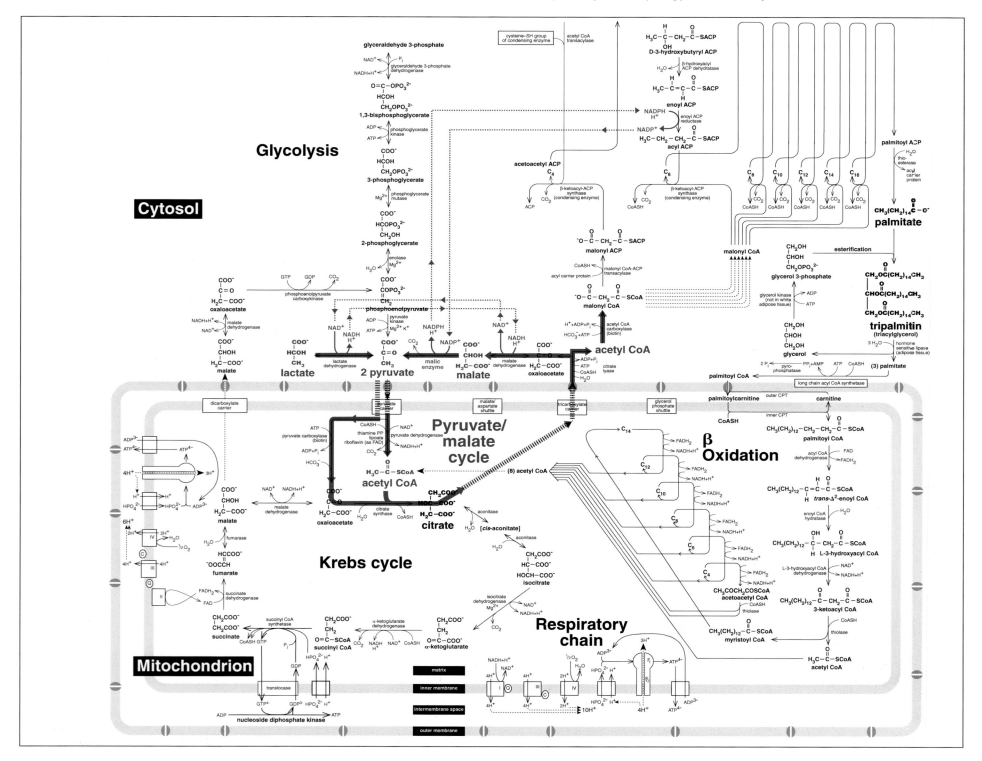

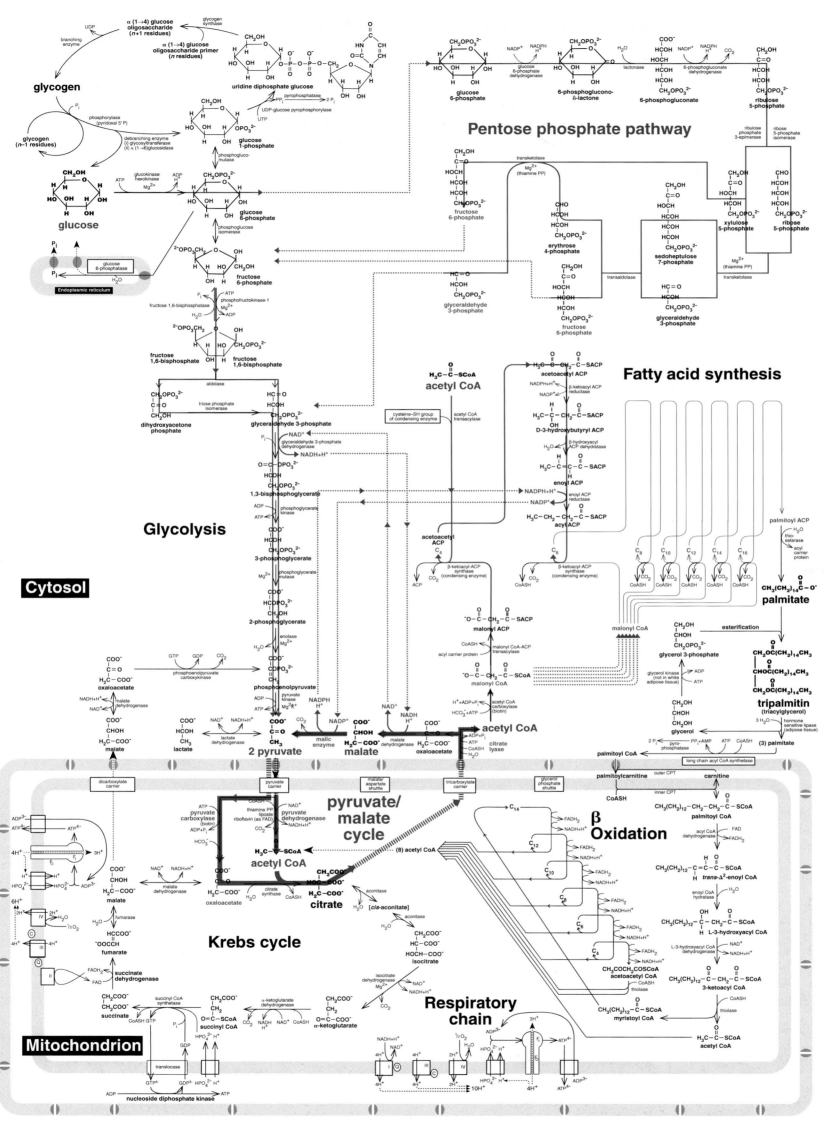

Chart 13.1 The pyruvate/malate cycle.

Mammals cannot synthesize glucose from fatty acids

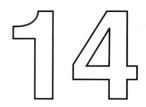

Fatty acids cannot be used as a gluconeogenic precursor by mammals for the reasons explained below. Since glucose is a vital fuel for brain and red blood cells, this presents a serious difficulty during prolonged starvation once the glycogen reserves have been depleted (although the brain can adapt to use ketone bodies as a respiratory fuel). It is unfortunate that, because the fatty acids derived from triacylglycerol in adipose tissue cannot be used for gluconeogenesis, muscle proteins must be degraded to maintain glucose homeostasis in the starving state, thereby causing wasting of the skeletal muscles.

Chart 14.1: In mammals, two molecules of carbon dioxide are evolved when acetyl CoA is oxidized in Krebs cycle

The chart illustrates why mammals cannot convert fatty acids to glucose. Fatty acids are oxidized to acetyl CoA. Because the pyruvate dehydrogenase

and pyruvate kinase reactions are irreversible, acetyl CoA cannot simply be carboxylated to pyruvate and proceed to form glucose by reversal of glycolysis. Instead, the two carbon atoms contained in the acetyl group of acetyl CoA enter Krebs cycle. However, two carbon atoms are removed as carbon dioxide as shown in the chart. Hence, in animals, there can be no **net** synthesis of glucose from acetyl CoA. Having emphasized this point, it should be noted that if fatty acids that are uniformly labelled with ^{14}C are fed to mammals, some of the radioactive label does become incorporated into glucose. This is because the ^{14}C-fatty acid is catabolized to ^{14}C-acetyl CoA, which enters Krebs cycle. The label is incorporated into citrate and may be retained in the other intermediates of the cycle. If ^{14}C-malate is formed, it can leave the mitochondrion and the ^{14}C label may be incorporated into glucose by gluconeogenesis. **NB:** This incorporation of ^{14}C-label from acetyl CoA into carbohydrate does not represent **net** synthesis because two carbon atoms have been lost as carbon dioxide in the process.

Glycerol derived from triacylglycerol can be used for glucose synthesis

When the triacylglycerol stored in adipose tissue is hydrolysed by hormone-sensitive lipase, fatty acids and glycerol are released. Unlike fatty acids, glycerol **can** be used for glucose synthesis by the liver (see Chapter 23). Glycerol is transported in the blood to the liver, where it is phosphorylated by **glycerol kinase** to glycerol 3-phosphate, which is reduced to dihydroxyacetone phosphate, two molecules of which are converted to glucose by gluconeogenesis, as shown in Chart 14.1.

Possible gluconeogenic pathways using fatty acid precursors in mammals

Draye and Vamecq have challenged the standard textbook dogma that mammals are unable to convert fatty acids to glucose. They point out that fatty acids with an odd number of carbon atoms, and branched-chain fatty acids, can be metabolized to produce succinyl CoA. Moreover, ω-oxidation of even-numbered fatty acids yields succinate. Both of these products are gluconeogenic precursors. However, gluconeogenesis from these fatty acids is unlikely to be quantitatively significant in physiological terms.

Chart 14.1 Two molecules of carbon dioxide are evolved when acetyl CoA is oxidized in Krebs cycle.

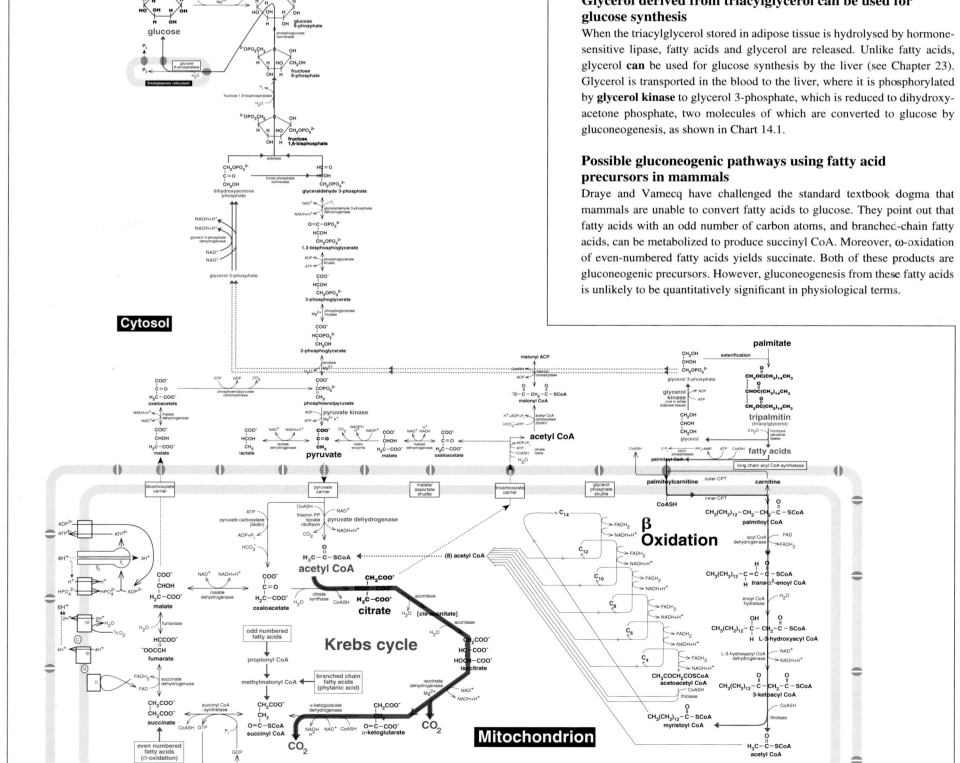

Chart 14.2 The glyoxylate cycle in plants.

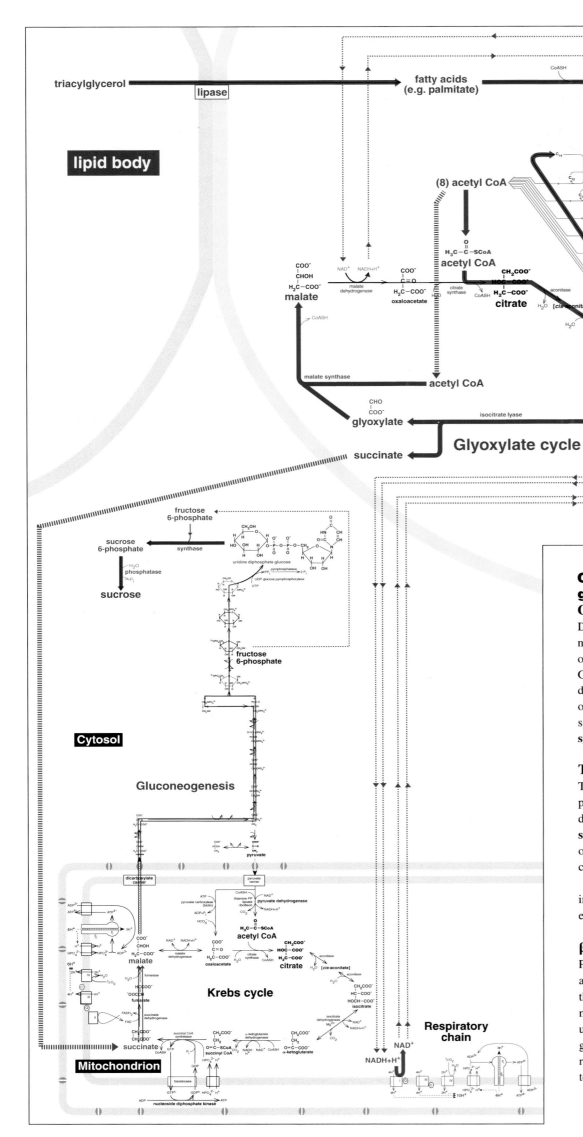

Chart 14.2: The glyoxylate cycle enables germinating seeds to synthesize sugars from fat

Glyoxysomes

During germination, oil-rich seeds can metabolize their stored fat to sugar, notably sucrose, for distribution throughout the developing seedling. This process occurs in specialized peroxisomes (or microbodies) known as glyoxysomes. Glyoxysomes are temporary organelles present for approximately one week during germination. Glyoxysomes contain all the enzymes for β-oxidation but only three of the Krebs cycle enzymes, namely malate dehydrogenase, citrate synthase and aconitase. In addition they contain **isocitrate lyase** and **malate synthase**, which enable 'the glyoxylate cycle' to proceed.

The glyoxylate cycle

The glyoxylate cycle resembles Krebs cycle, with some notable differences. In particular, the CO_2-losing stages of the latter (the isocitrate and α-ketoglutarate dehydrogenases) are absent. Instead, **isocitrate lyase** forms **glyoxylate** and **succinate**. Succinate leaves the glyoxysome, enters the mitochondrion and is oxidized to **malate**. The latter leaves the mitochondrion to form sucrose in the cytosol.

Meanwhile, back in the glyoxysome, the glyoxylate combines with acetyl CoA in the presence of malate synthase to produce malate, with is oxidized to oxaloacetate, thereby completing the cycle.

β-Oxidation in plants

Plant mitochondria generally lack the enyzmes needed for the β-oxidation of fatty acids. Instead, fatty acids are oxidized in peroxisomes (glyoxysomes of seeds). In these organelles the first oxidation reaction, catalysed by **acyl CoA oxidase**, uses molecular oxygen and produces hydrogen peroxide (see Chart 14.2). It is not fully understood how reoxidation of the NADH formed by β-oxidation and the glyoxylate cycle occurs. It has been suggested that glyoxysomes have a rudimentary electron transport chain. Alternatively, NADH could be transported to the mitochondrion as shown.

Metabolism of triacylglycerol to provide energy as ATP

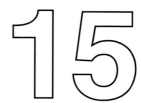

Fatty acids are oxidized and ATP is formed

Fatty acids are esterified with glycerol to form triacylglycerols, which are stored in adipose tissue. They are an important respiratory fuel for many tissues, especially muscle. The complete oxidation of a typical fatty acid, palmitate, is shown in Chart 15.1.

Chart 15.1: The oxidation of fatty acids with energy conserved as ATP

Three metabolic pathways are involved. These are: the **β-oxidation pathway,** Krebs cycle and the **respiratory chain**. First of all, **hormone-sensitive lipase** in adipose tissue must liberate fatty acids from **triacylglycerol**. The chart shows the hydrolysis of the triacylglycerol tripalmitin to yield three molecules of **palmitate** and one molecule of **glycerol**. Next, **palmitoyl CoA** is formed in a reaction catalysed by **long chain acyl CoA synthetase**; ATP is consumed in the process and AMP (adenosine monophosphate) and inorganic pyrophosphate (PP$_i$) are formed. Thus energy equal to two ATP equivalents is required for this activation reaction. The palmitoyl CoA formed is transported into the mitochondrion using the carnitine shuttle (Chapter 26). Once in the mitochondrial matrix it is successively oxidized and cleaved to yield eight 2-carbon fragments of acetyl CoA by the β-oxidation pathway. For each turn of the β-oxidation cycle, one FADH$_2$ and one NADH are formed, thus seven FADH$_2$ and seven NADH are formed from palmitate. The eight molecules of acetyl CoA then enter Krebs cycle, where they are oxidized as shown. The ATP yield using the 'modern' non-integral values for the P/O ratios is as follows: the NADH and FADH$_2$ formed by both β-oxidation and Krebs cycle are oxidized by the respiratory chain and yield a total of 100 ATP by oxidative phosphorylation. A further net gain of six ATP is derived from the eight GTP molecules produced by substrate-level phosphorylation in Krebs cycle.

By inspecting Chart 15.1, we can now take stock of the ATP net yield from one molecule of palmitate (see Table 15.1 opposite).

For comparison, the ATP net yield from palmitate using the traditional integral values for P/O ratios is shown in Table 15.2.

Table 15.2 The traditional method for calculating ATP net yield from palmitate (see Chapter 6, Chart 6.1).

From β-oxidation	ATP yield
By oxidative phosphorylation of 7 FADH$_2$	14
By oxidative phosphorylation of 7 NADH	21
	35 ATP

From Krebs cycle	ATP yield
By substrate-level phosphorylation via GTP	8
By oxidative phosphorylation of 8 FADH$_2$	16
By oxidative phosphorylation of 24 NADH	72
	96 ATP

The total yield is therefore 35+96=131 ATP. We must remember, however, to subtract the two ATP equivalents consumed in the initial acyl CoA synthetase reaction. **Therefore the net yield from the oxidation of one molecule of palmitate is 129 molecules of ATP.**

triacylglycerol

glycerol ←

hormone
sensitive
lipase

adipocyte

fatty acids

fatty acids to
muscle for use as
a respiratory fuel

fatty acids

sarcolemma

sarcoplasm

mitochondrion

β-oxidation

8 acetyl
CoA

myofibril

Diagram 15.1 When energy is required under conditions of stress such as 'fight or flight', exercise or starvation, the hormones adrenaline and glucagon stimulate triacylglycerol mobilization by activating hormone-sensitive lipase in adipose tissue (Chapter 25), and fatty acids and glycerol are released. The fatty acids are bound to albumin and transported in the blood to the tissues for oxidation, e.g. by muscle. The glycerol is converted by the liver to glucose (Chapter 23), which in turn is released for oxidation, especially by the red blood cells and brain, neither of which can use fatty acids as a respiratory fuel.

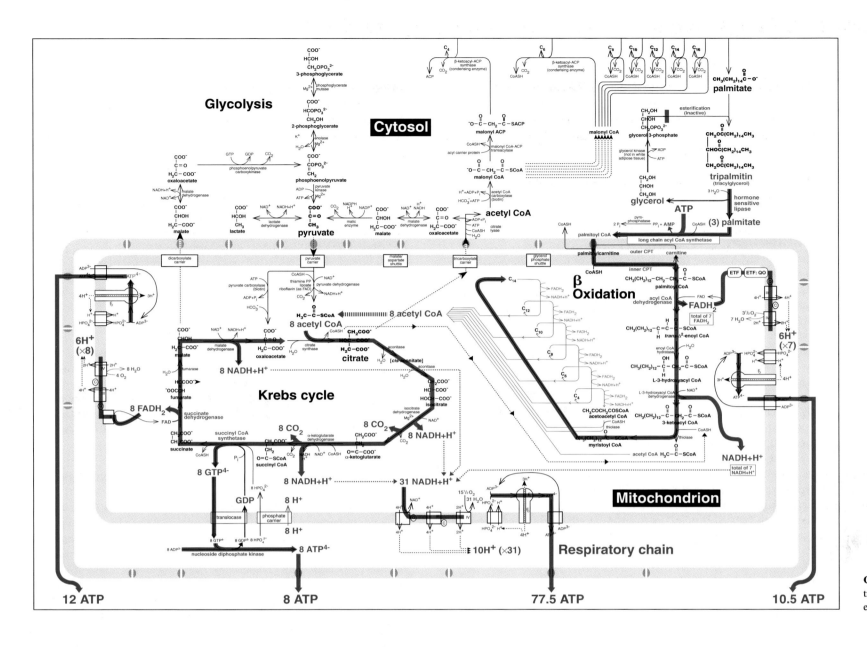

Chart 15.1 Metabolism of triacylglycerol to provide energy as ATP.

Table 15.1 ATP net yield from the oxidation of hexadecanoate (palmitate) assuming non-integral values for P/O ratios (see Chapter 6, Chart 6.2).

Origin	Mechanism	Number of protons	ATP yield (loss)
Mitochondrion 31 molecules of NADH	*Oxidative phophorylation* The β-oxidation spiral and Krebs cycle yield 31 molecules of NADH which, when oxidized, provide energy to pump 31×10 protons (i.e. 310). Since four protons are used to synthesize and translocate one ATP, therefore $310 \div 4 = 77.5$ ATP are made	310	**77.5 ATP**
Acyl CoA dehydrogenase forms 7 FADH$_2$	Acyl CoA dehydrogenase forms 7 FADH$_2$ which, when oxidized, provide energy to pump 7×6 (i.e. 42 protons). Since four protons are used to synthesize and translocate one ATP, therefore $42 \div 4 = 10.5$ molecules of ATP are made	42	**10.5 ATP**
Succinate dehydrogenase forms 8 FADH$_2$	Succinate dehydrogenase forms 8 FADH$_2$ which provides energy to pump 8×6 (i.e. 48 protons) from the matrix, equivalent to the formation of $48 \div 4 = 12$ ATP	48	**12 ATP**
Mitochondrion Succinyl CoA synthetase forms 8 GTP	*Substrate-level phosphorylation* 8 GTP yield 8 ATP in the nucleoside diphosphate kinase reaction		**8 ATP**
Phosphate carrier	Phosphate/proton symport. Import of 8 phosphate anions uses 8 protons from the electrochemical gradient (equivalent to losing 2 ATP)	−8	**(−2 ATP)**
Cytosol Acyl CoA synthetase	*Activation of fatty acids* Acyl CoA synthetase uses ATP and forms AMP and pyrophosphate. This is equivalent to the loss of 2 molecules of ATP forming ADP		**(−2 ATP)**
		ATP net yield from oxidation of palmitate	**104 ATP**

Glycogen metabolism I

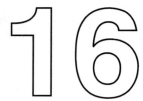

The different roles of glycogen in liver and muscle

Although both liver and muscle store glycogen, there are major differences between the two in the way that glycogen metabolism is deployed and controlled. The liver exports glucose derived from glycogen for use by other tissues. In skeletal muscle, the glucose is particularly important as a fuel, one that is immediately available during periods of extreme activity, such as in the adrenaline-driven 'fight or flight' response.

The metabolic demands made on glycogen metabolism

The simplistic approach to glycogen metabolism is to consider glycogen synthesis in the fed state, followed by glycogen breakdown during fasting or 'fight or flight', followed by glycogen synthesis after feeding to complete the cycle. However, nature does not order periods of feeding, fasting and fight or flight with carefully planned transition periods in between. Indeed, in nature, animals are very vulnerable to attack by a predator when they are feeding. The prey's muscles must then respond to the crisis by instantly diverting the flux of glucose metabolites from the feeding state of glycogen **synthesis** to glycogen **breakdown** for anaerobic glycolysis. Furthermore, this instantaneous metabolic U-turn must be achieved in spite of the lingering presence of insulin secreted during feeding, which tends to promote glycogen synthesis. Next, after a strenuous chase, the prey (assuming it has survived) must quickly replenish its glycogen reserves for the next emergency, whether food is available or not. Moreover, this must be done without excessively draining blood glucose concentrations and causing hypoglycaemia. Not surprisingly, the complicated physiological demands made on glycogen metabolism are matched by a complicated regulatory mechanism. The details of this mechanism are still not fully understood, but it involves an **amplification cascade** dramatically enhancing the effects of the hormones that initiate this series of reactions (see Chapter 17).

Glycogen metabolism: an overview

Liver and muscle share some general features during the processes of glycogen synthesis from glucose 1-phosphate, and glycogenolysis back to glucose 1-phosphate; these are summarized below.

Glycogenesis

Glucose 1-phosphate reacts with **uridine triphosphate (UTP)** (see Chart 16.2) to form **uridine diphosphate glucose (UDP-glucose)**. This is an activated form of glucose used for glycogen synthesis. A **primer**, in the form of an $\alpha(1\rightarrow4)$-glucose oligosaccharide attached to the protein glycogenin, is also needed. The glucosyl group from UDP-glucose is added to the polysaccharide chain by **glycogen synthase** provided it consists of four or more glucose residues. Once the chain contains 11 or more residues, the **branching enzyme** becomes involved. The branching enzyme forms the many branches of glycogen by severing a string of seven residues from the growing chain and rejoining it by an $\alpha(1\rightarrow6)$-linkage to an interior point at least four residues from an existing branch.

Glycogenolysis

The enzyme controlling glycogenolysis is **phosphorylase** (see Chart 16.1). It requires pyridoxal phosphate and inorganic phosphate and exists in both active and inactive forms. Phosphorylase progressively nibbles its way along the chain of $\alpha(1\rightarrow4)$-glucose molecules, releasing molecules of **glucose 1-phosphate**. Its progress is obstructed when it reaches a stage on the chain four glucose residues away from a branch point. Now the bifunctional debranching enzyme is needed, one component of which, **glycosyltransferase**, rescues the situation by transferring the terminal three (of these four) glucose molecules to the end of another chain so that phosphorylase activity can continue. The remaining glucose molecule, which now forms an $\alpha(1\rightarrow6)$-linked stump at the branching point, is removed as free glucose by $\alpha(1\rightarrow6)$-**glucosidase**, the second component of the debranching enzyme.

The glucose 1-phosphate formed by phosphorylase is converted to glucose 6-phosphate by phosphoglucomutase.

Glycogen metabolism in liver

The liver stores glycogen as a reserve fuel for periods of fasting or 'fight or flight'. Liver does not usually use the glycogen-derived glucose itself for energy; instead it is exported for use by the brain, erythrocytes and muscle.

Glycogenolysis in liver

Glycogenolysis (see Chart 16.1) is stimulated by glucagon in response to fasting, and by adrenaline for 'fight or flight'. Both of these hormones stimulate the **glycogenolysis cascade** (see Diagram 17.1) to produce glucose 6-phosphate. Liver (unlike muscle) has **glucose 6-phosphatase**, which enables mobilization of glucose into the blood.

NB: In liver, in contrast to muscle, cyclic AMP-mediated phosphorylation **inhibits** glycolysis and stimulates hepatic gluconeogenesis (see Chapter 20). In the physiological context this means that during fasting, when glucagon is present, both glycogenolysis and gluconeogenesis will be active.

Glycogen synthesis in liver
Glycogenesis: the 'direct' pathway from dietary glucose

Traditionally it was thought that glucose from dietary carbohydrate is transported **directly** to the liver for metabolism to glycogen, i.e. by the '**direct pathway**' for glycogenesis (see Chart 16.2). However, evidence suggests that following a fast, during the period immediately after refeeding, glycogen synthesis proceeds via an '**indirect pathway**' involving skeletal muscle (see below).

Glycogenesis: the 'indirect' pathway from dietary glucose via muscle lactate

During refeeding after fasting, glucose is metabolized anaerobically to lactate by muscle even though the conditions are aerobic. This is because, immediately after refeeding, the high ratio of acetyl CoA/CoA caused by the lingering β-oxidation of fatty acids, results in pyruvate dehydrogenase remaining inhibited (see Chapter 38). Consequently, glucose in muscle is metabolized to pyruvate, which is reduced to lactate. This lactate is transported in the blood to the liver for gluconeogenesis and glycogen synthesis.

Liver glycogen storage diseases
Type I glycogen storage disease (von Gierke's disease)

In Type I glycogen storage disease (GSD), glycogen accumulates in the liver, kidneys and intestines. It has been divided into subtypes, of which types Ia, Ib and Ic are shown in Chart 16.3. The basic defect is glucose 6-phosphatase deficiency either from loss of the catalytic enzyme unit itself (Ia), or of either the endoplasmic reticulum glucose 6-phosphate translocator (Ib) or the phosphate translocator (Ic) (see also Diagram 23.1).

In all cases the clinical features are identical and are a consequence of the substrate cycling of glucose 6-phosphate shown in Chart 16.3. Patients have low levels of blood glucose, and raised levels of lactate, ketone bodies, lipids and urate. Lactate supplied by the extrahepatic tissues is metabolized to glucose 6-phosphate. In the absence of glucose 6-phosphatase, it cannot be metabolized to glucose resulting in hypoglycaemia, which is potentially fatal. Instead, it is diverted into glycogen synthesis causing hepatomegaly, and into the pentose phosphate pathway forming ribose 5-phosphate, which is a precursor of purine synthesis. Purine catabolism forms uric acid, which can cause gout.

Type VI glycogen storage disease (Hers' disease)

This condition is due to deficiency of liver phosphorylase (or phosphorylase kinase) as shown in Chart 16.1. Similarly to Type I disease, this causes hepatomegaly due to glycogen accumulation. However, because normal blood glucose levels can be maintained by gluconeogenesis from lactate, alanine, glycerol, etc., ketosis is moderate and hyperlactataemia does not occur.

Type III debranching enzyme deficiency (Cori's disease)

Patients are deficient in $\alpha(1\rightarrow6)$-glucosidase (AGL) activity and present with hypoglycaemia and hyperlipidaemia (see Chart 16.1). Usually, both liver and muscle AGL is affected (subtype IIIa) but, in 15% of cases, the muscle enzyme is intact while the liver enzyme is deficient (subtype IIIb).

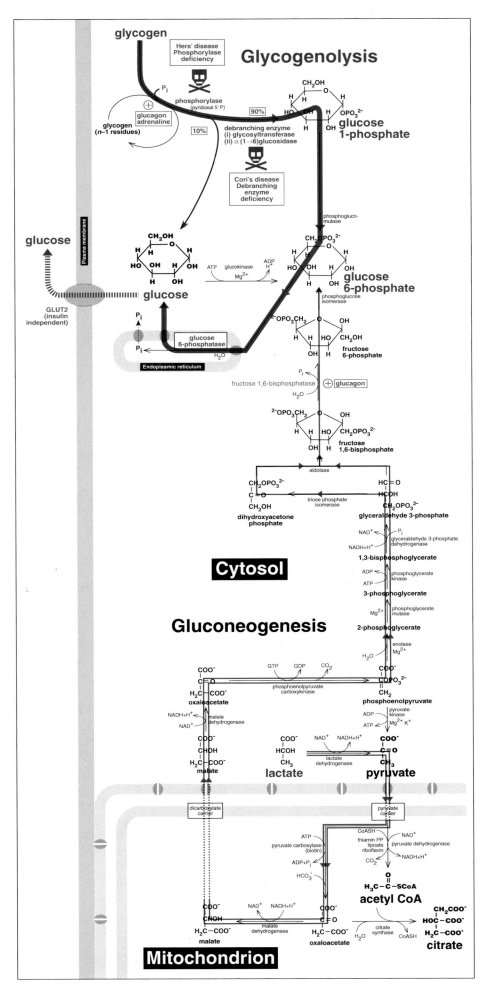

Chart 16.1 Glycogenolysis in liver.

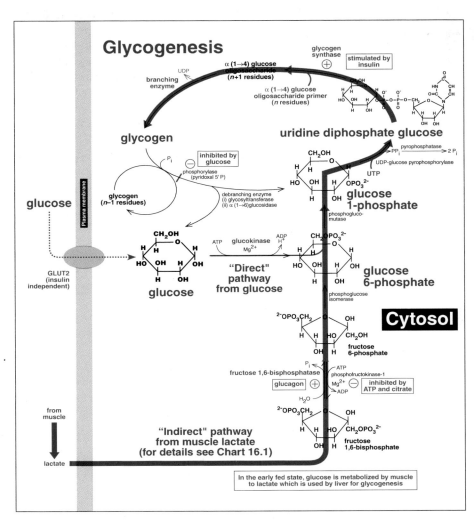

Chart 16.2 Glycogenesis in liver from glucose (direct pathway), and from lactate (indirect pathway).

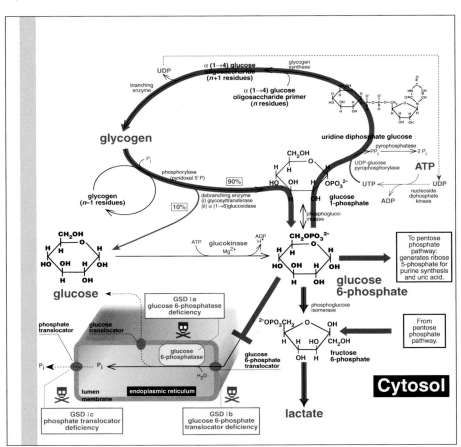

Chart 16.3 Glycogenolysis in Type I glycogen storage disease.

Glycogen metabolism II

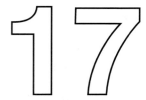

Glycogen metabolism in skeletal muscle

In muscle, the main function of glycogen is to serve as a reserve of respiratory fuel by rapidly providing glucose during periods of extremely vigorous muscle contraction, such as occur in moments of danger, i.e. in the 'fight or flight' response.

Glycogenolysis in skeletal muscle

Glycogenolysis in skeletal muscle (see Chart 17.1) is stimulated by adrenaline via the amplification cascade shown in Diagram 17.1. **Phosphorylase** produces **glucose 1-phosphate**, which is converted into **glucose 6-phosphate**. Because muscle lacks glucose 6-phosphatase, glucose 6-phosphate is totally committed to glycolysis for ATP production. Also, since muscle hexokinase has a very low K_m for glucose (0.1 mmol/l), it has a very high affinity for glucose and will readily phosphorylate the 10% of glucose units liberated from glycogen by the debranching enzyme, $\alpha(1\rightarrow6)$-glucosidase, as free glucose, thus ensuring its use by glycolysis. It should be remembered that adrenaline increases the cyclic AMP concentration, which not only stimulates glycogenolysis but **in muscle** also stimulates glycolysis (see Chapter 20).

Glycogen synthesis in skeletal muscle

In the fed state in resting muscle, insulin is available to facilitate glucose transport into the muscle cell using the GLUT4 transporter (see Chart 17.2). Remember that, in the fed state, phosphofructokinase-1 is inhibited (see Chapter 20) and so glucose 6-phosphate will be used for glycogen synthesis. It should be noted that glycogen synthesis and glycogenolysis are regulated in a reciprocal way (see Diagram 17.1).

The glycogenolysis cascade

Diagram 17.1 shows how the original signal provided by a single molecule of adrenaline is amplified during the course of a cascade of reactions that activate a large number of phosphorylase molecules, ensuring the rapid mobilization of glycogen as follows:

1 A molecule of adrenaline stimulates adenylate cyclase to form several molecules of **cyclic AMP**.
2 Each molecule of cyclic AMP dissociates an inactive tetramer to free two catalytically active monomers of **protein kinase A** (also known as **cyclic AMP-dependent protein kinase**) from their regulatory monomers. **NB:** This gives a relatively modest amplification factor of two.
3 Each active molecule of protein kinase A phosphorylates and activates several molecules of **phosphorylase kinase**.

At this point, reciprocal regulation of glycogen synthesis and breakdown occurs. First, let us continue with glycogenolysis before concluding with the inactivation of glycogen synthesis.

4 One molecule of phosphorylase kinase phosphorylates several inactive molecules of **phosphorylase b** to give the active form, **phosphorylase a**, and so glycogen breakdown can now proceed.

Inactivation of glycogen synthesis

To maximize glycogen breakdown, synthesis is reciprocally inactivated by phosphorylase kinase, which is one of several protein kinases, including protein kinase A, which can cause **glycogen synthase a** to produce its low-activity **synthase b** form (see Diagram 17.1).

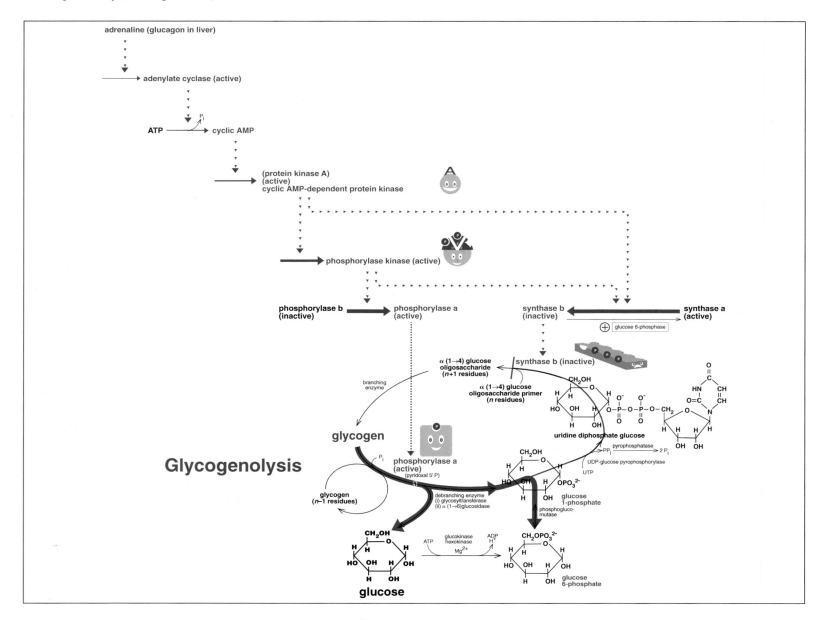

Diagram 17.1 Activation of the glycogenolysis cascade is linked to the inactivation of glycogen synthesis.

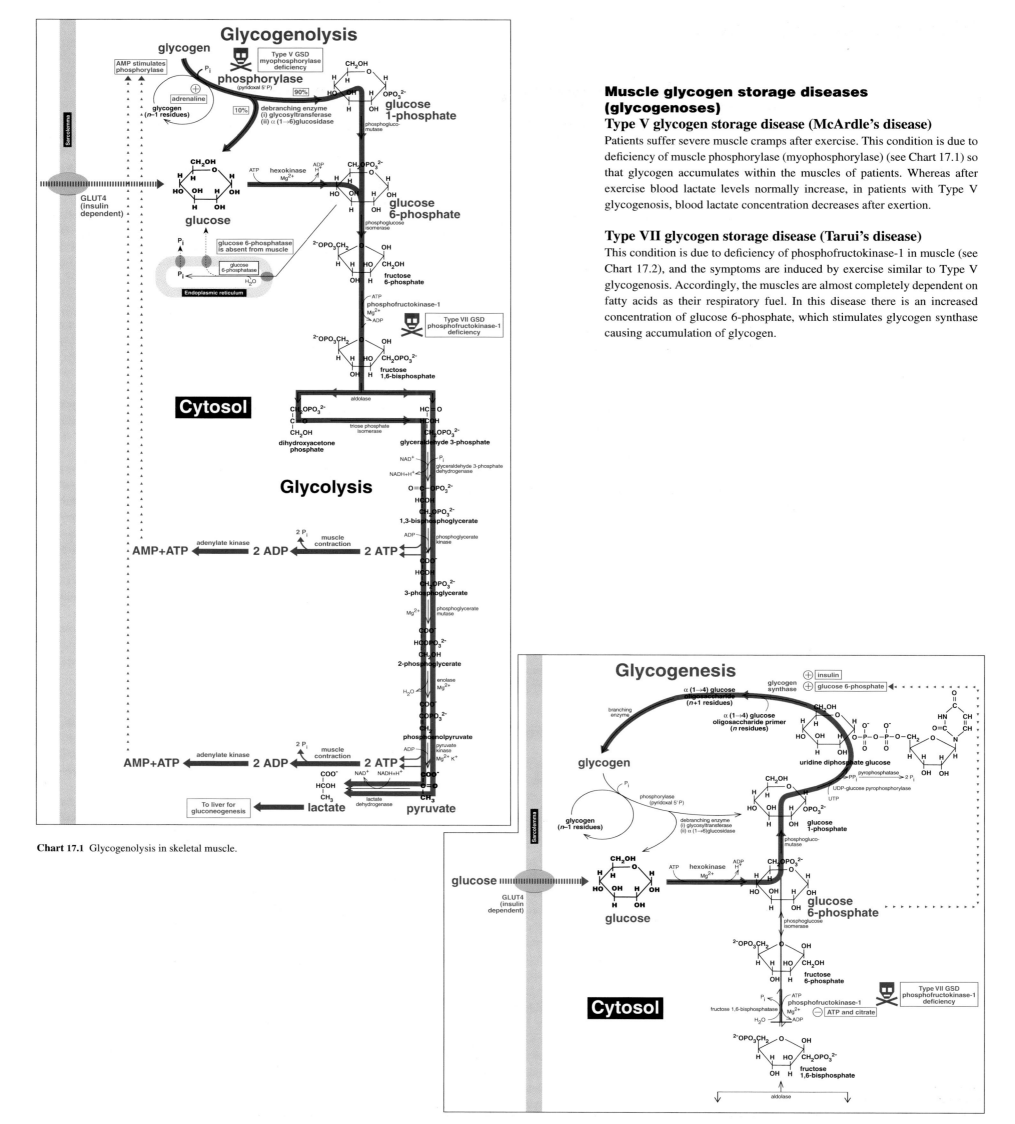

Chart 17.1 Glycogenolysis in skeletal muscle.

Chart 17.2 Glycogenesis in skeletal muscle.

Muscle glycogen storage diseases (glycogenoses)

Type V glycogen storage disease (McArdle's disease)

Patients suffer severe muscle cramps after exercise. This condition is due to deficiency of muscle phosphorylase (myophosphorylase) (see Chart 17.1) so that glycogen accumulates within the muscles of patients. Whereas after exercise blood lactate levels normally increase, in patients with Type V glycogenosis, blood lactate concentration decreases after exertion.

Type VII glycogen storage disease (Tarui's disease)

This condition is due to deficiency of phosphofructokinase-1 in muscle (see Chart 17.2), and the symptoms are induced by exercise similar to Type V glycogenosis. Accordingly, the muscles are almost completely dependent on fatty acids as their respiratory fuel. In this disease there is an increased concentration of glucose 6-phosphate, which stimulates glycogen synthase causing accumulation of glycogen.

Glycogen metabolism III: regulation of glycogen breakdown

18

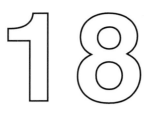

Diagram 18.1 (opposite) Regulation of glycogenolysis.

Hormonal control: the role of adrenaline and glucagon in the regulation of glycogenolysis

In liver, glycogenolysis is stimulated by both glucagon and adrenaline, whereas in muscle only adrenaline is effective. In a crisis, when mobilization of glycogen is stimulated by adrenaline, the response must happen **immediately!** This occurs through the remarkable amplification cascade described earlier (see Chapter 17), in which cyclic AMP plays an important role. In this way, small, nanomolar concentrations of adrenaline can rapidly mobilize a vast number of glucose residues for use as respiratory fuel.

NB: The regulation of glycogen metabolism, which is complex, is still the subject of extensive research and full details are beyond the scope of this book (see Chapter 50). **The descriptions provided here and in the next chapter are based on current knowledge, largely relating to the regulation of glycogen metabolism in skeletal muscle.** *Whereas many details of the mechanisms may be common to both liver and muscle, there are several differences stemming from the different functions of the two tissues; for example, whereas both liver and muscle are responsive to adrenaline (albeit through different mechanisms), only liver has receptors for glucagon.*

Diagram 18.1: Regulation of glycogenolysis
Formation of cyclic AMP

When adrenaline docks with its receptor in muscle, the signal is transduced through the G protein, **adenylate cylase** is activated, and ATP is converted to **cyclic AMP,** which activates **protein kinase A.**

Protein kinase A (also known as cyclic AMP-dependent protein kinase)

When inactive, protein kinase A exists as part of a tetramer consisting of two catalytic subunits and two regulatory (R) subunits (see Diagram 18.2). When cyclic AMP is present, it binds to the two regulatory units and liberates the two active catalytic subunits.

NB: These active monomers of protein kinase A (and their metabolic opponents, the protein phosphatases, described more fully in the next chapter) play a key role in regulating not only glycogen metabolism, but also many other pathways of intermediary metabolism (see Chapters 20, 23 & 25).

Returning to glycogen metabolism, protein kinase A plays a major role in both **activating** glycogenolysis and concurrently enhancing this function by **inhibiting** glycogen synthesis.

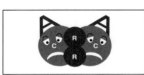

Diagram 18.2 Inactive protein kinase A.

Roles of protein kinase A in regulating glycogenolysis

Protein kinase A phosphorylates several enzymes involved in glycogen metabolism, and these covalent modifications persist until the enzymes are dephosphorylated by protein phosphatases (see Chapter 19). The effects of protein kinase A, shown in the diagram opposite, are:

1 **Activation of phosphorylase kinase.** Protein kinase A phosphorylates phosphorylase kinase to yield the active form. However, full activity requires Ca^{2+} ions, which are released into the sarcoplasm when muscle is contracting (or following α-adrenergic stimulation of liver). The fully activated phosphorylase kinase now has a double action: not only does it activate phosphorylase by forming **phosphorylase a** (see Diagram 18.1), but it also participates in phosphorylating (and thus inactivating) glycogen synthase.

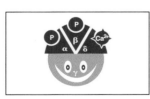

Diagram 18.3 Very active phosphorylase kinase.

2 **Inactivation of protein phosphatase-1.** Protein phosphatase-1 (see Chapter 19) plays a major role in switching off glycogenolysis by converting phosphorylase a (the active form) to the inactive phosphorylase b. Clearly this must be stopped. Accordingly, protein phosphatase-1 is inactivated by two assassins in the forms of protein kinase A and the **protein phosphatase inhibitor-1** (see section below). The first attack is by protein kinase A, which phosphorylates site 2 of the regulatory subunit of the protein phosphatase-1G complex. The consequence of this covalent modification is that protein phosphatase-1 dissociates from its sanctuary in the complex. The free protein phosphatase-1 is relatively inactive. Moreover, it is now unprotected and vulnerable to a second attack by the protein phosphatase inhibitor-1, which diffuses into action and delivers the *coup de grâce.*

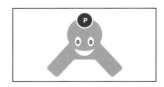

Diagram 18.4 Active protein phosphatase inhibitor-1.

So, finally, with the counterproductive interference by protein phosphatase-1 activity well and truly suppressed, phosphorylase a activity prevails unchallenged and glycogen breakdown can now take place.

3 **Activation of the protein phosphatase inhibitor-1.** The conspiracy between protein kinase A and the protein phosphatase inhibitor-1 is initiated when the latter is phosphorylated to its active form by the former. The active inhibitor can now join protein kinase A in the vendetta against protein phosphatase, as described in item 2 above.

4 **Resumption of glycogen synthesis after 'fight or flight'.** Rapid replacement of the glycogen stores is needed after a 'fight or flight' incident to survive the next crisis. Furthermore, this must be accomplished in the absence of insulin. Protein kinase A fulfils this requirement by phosphorylating **both** sites 1 and 2 of the regulatory subunit G thereby inactivating protein phosphatase-1 during the emergency. However, during recovery when adrenaline stimulation has finished, site 2 is preferentially dephosphorylated. This leaves site 1 phosphorylated and protein phosphatase-1 active and immediately able to activate glycogen synthase (see Diagram 19.1).

Phosphorylase kinase

This is a large 1300 kDa protein and is a hexadecamer of four subunits (see Diagram 18.3), each subunit being a tetramer of α-, β-, γ- and δ-monomers; the native protein thus comprises $\alpha_4\beta_4\gamma_4\delta_4$. The catalytic site is on the γ-monomer.

The α- and β-monomers are phosphorylated during modification from the inactive b form to the active phosphorylase kinase a. Although phosphorylation of the α-monomer causes some stimulation of activity, it is the subsequent rapid phosphorylation of the β-monomer that is the major activator of phosphorylase kinase activity. The δ-monomer is composed of calmodulin, which has four regulatory binding sites with different affinities for calcium ions. They can bind calcium ions at concentrations as low as $0.1\,\mu mol/l$, such as occur in resting muscle. However, they are fully occupied and maximally stimulated following the 100-fold increase in calcium ion concentration – up to $10\,\mu mol/l$ – that occurs during exercise.

Phosphorylase kinase a is inhibited when it is dephosphorylated by **protein phosphatase-1**, which removes phosphate from the β-monomer, and by **protein phosphatase-2A**, which demodifies the α-monomer (see Diagram 19.1).

Properties of glycogen phosphorylase

Phosphorylase b is a dimer of two identical 97 kDa proteins, which are associated with glycogen and can be phosphorylated at the serine residue at N-14 by phosphorylase kinase to form **phosphorylase a.** The latter is a tetramer formed by dimerization of phosphorylase b (for simplicity, the monomer is shown in the diagram opposite).

In resting muscle, phosphorylase b is in the inactive T form; in contracting muscle it is in the active R form. During exercise, ATP is converted to AMP. The increase in AMP concentration stimulates phosphorylase b by forming the R form, which decreases its K_m for phosphate. Conversely, ATP and glucose 6-phosphate counter the effect of AMP so that in the resting state, as the concentrations of the former recover, phosphorylase b is converted back to the inactive T form.

Phosphorylase a is not dependent on AMP for activity, provided the concentration of P_i is sufficiently increased, as happens during muscle contraction. It is formed by the action of phosphorylase kinase, as described above, and undergoes a conformational change from the T form to the active R form.

Inactivation of phosphorylase a is by demodification by protein phosphatase-1 (see Diagram 19.1).

Protein phosphatase inhibitor-1

The inhibitor-1 is an 18.7 kDa protein that is modified to its active form by phosphorylation of a threonine residue in a reaction catalysed by protein kinase A (see Diagram 18.4). The inhibitor inactivates protein phosphatase-1 but has no effect on protein phosphatase-2A. In resting muscle, i.e. when glycogenolysis is not active, protein phosphatase inhibitor-1 is inactivated when it is dephosphorylated by protein phosphatase-2A (see Diagram 19.1).

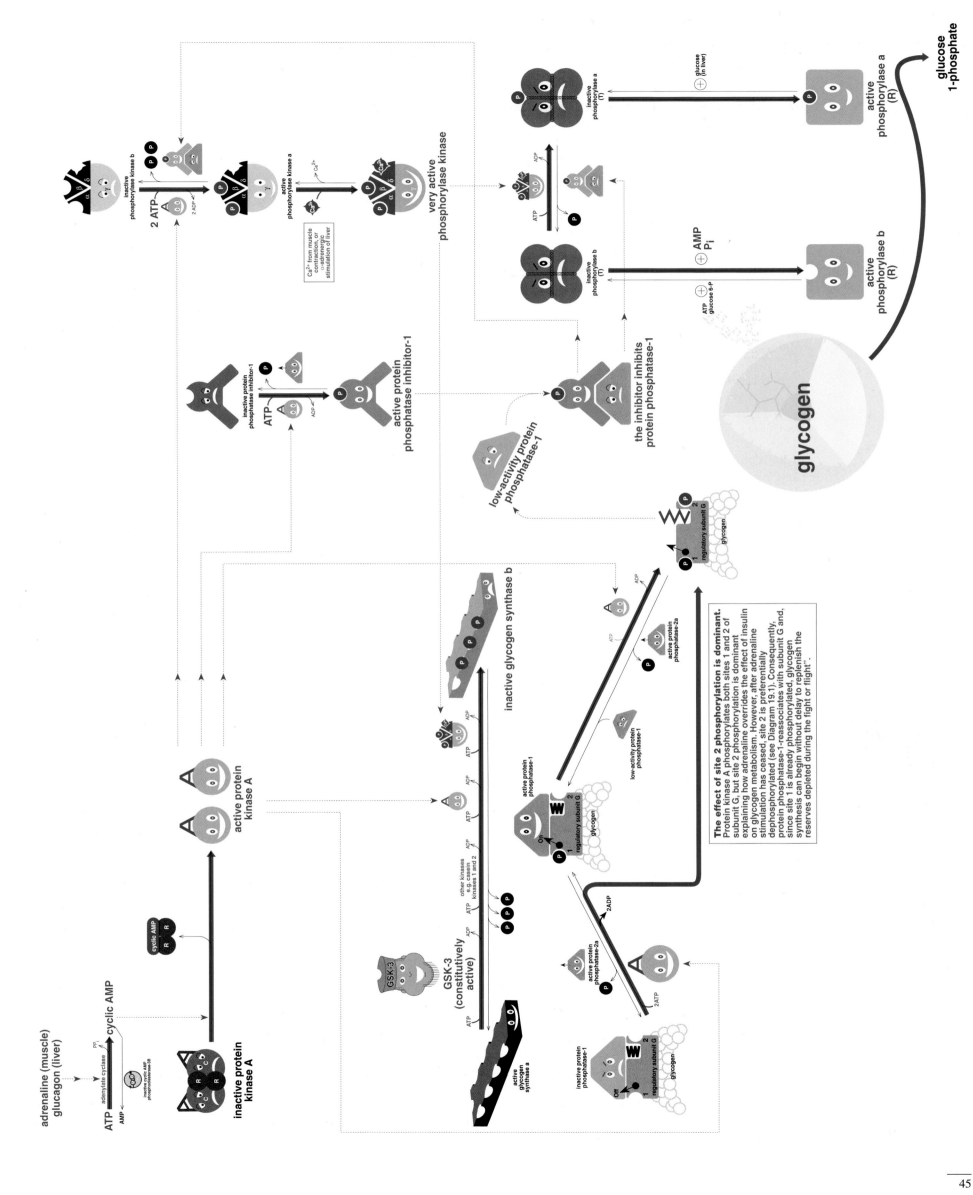

Glycogen metabolism IV: regulation of glycogen synthesis

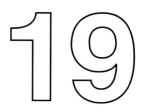

Hormonal control: the role of insulin in the regulation of glycogen synthesis

Insulin is secreted by the β-cells of the pancreas following a carbohydrate meal. Insulin is needed to transport glucose into muscle cells, which means that glycogenesis is most active in the post-prandial state. Having stressed the importance of insulin in regulating glycogen synthesis, it is something of an anticlimax to confess that many details of insulin action are imperfectly understood, in spite of much recent progress (see Chapter 50). However, fundamental to glycogen synthesis is the regulation of **glycogen synthase**, which is regulated as shown in Diagrams 18.1 and 19.1.

Diagram 19.1 (opposite)
Regulation of glycogenesis.

*Glycogen synthesis has been studied most extensively in muscle, and it is to this tissue that the following description of regulation relates. It should be noted that, whereas in the catabolic state of glycogenolysis, phosphorylation by protein kinases dominates the scene, in the anabolic state of glycogenesis, the **protein phosphatases -1** and **-2A** dominate and protein dephosphorylation occurs.*

Protein phosphatases

Protein phosphatase-1 and protein phosphatase-2A are the protein phosphatases in skeletal muscle that are involved in the regulation of glycogen metabolism.

Protein phosphatase-1 (PP-1)

Experiments suggest that this is a 37 kDa protein. It is inhibited by inhibitor-1 and by okadaic acid. There are several forms of PP-1, but the major active form associated with glycogen is known as PP-1G. This is a complex of PP-1 and a large, 160 kDa regulatory subunit G, which is bound to glycogen.

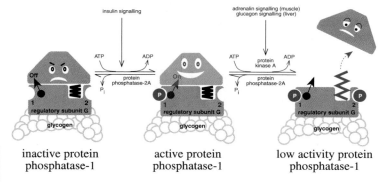

inactive protein phosphatase-1   active protein phosphatase-1   low activity protein phosphatase-1

Regulation of PP-1G activity

PP-1G is active when phosphorylated at site 1 by insulin-generated signals via phosphatidylinositol-3 kinase (PI-3 kinase) (Chapter 50). Conversely, it is slowly inactivated by dephosphorylation of site 1 by protein phosphatase-2A. However, PP-1 is also inactivated by phosphorylation at site 2 by protein kinase A, which causes the catalytic subunit to dissociate from the regulatory subunit G. The latter process is reversed by protein phosphatase-2A, which dephosphorylates site 2 permitting reassociation of the subunits to form active PP-1G.

Protein phosphatase-2A (PP-2A)

Several forms of PP-2A have been identified in eukaryotic cells, some containing two subunits and some three subunits. It is inhibited by okadaic acid but is not inhibited by inhibitor-1 (see Diagram 19.2).

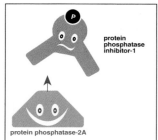

Diagram 19.2 Protein phosphatase-2A is not inhibited by protein phosphatase inhibitor-1.

Diagram 19.1: Regulation of glycogen synthesis
Removal of cyclic AMP

We have seen in the previous chapter how hormone-stimulated mobilization of glycogen is mediated by cyclic AMP. Obviously, if glycogen synthesis is to occur glycogen breakdown must stop, and so cyclic AMP must be destroyed. There is evidence based on studies of adipose tissue suggesting the presence of an insulin-stimulated series of reactions that results in the activation of **cyclic AMP phosphodiesterase-3B (PDE-3B)** and conversion of cyclic AMP to AMP (Diagram 54.1).

Diagram 19.3 Active glycogen synthase a.

Role of protein phosphatase-1 and -2A in regulating glycogenesis

With PP-1 active, glycogen synthesis can begin in earnest. Basically, PP-1 and PP-2A oppose the action of the protein kinases and they have the following effects:

1 **Inactivation of PP-1 inhibitor.** In resting muscle, PP-2A inactivates the **PP-1** inhibitor in an act of biochemical camaraderie that is much appreciated by its team mate, PP-1.
2 **Inactivation of phosphorylase kinase.** PP-1 dephosphorylates the β-monomer, and PP-2A dephosphorylates the α-monomer, thereby inactivating **phosphorylase kinase**. This prevents the formation of **phosphorylase a** thus inhibiting glycogen breakdown.
3 **Activation of glycogen synthase.** Finally, PP-1 dephosphorylates **synthase b** to form the high-activity **synthase a**, which catalyses the formation of glycogen from uridine diphosphate glucose.

Properties of glycogen synthase

Glycogen synthase is a simple tetramer of four identical 85 kDa monomers (for simplicity, a single monomer is shown in Diagram 19.3). Its activity is regulated by synergistic phosphorylation, which can occur at nine sites (serine residues) in a precise, hierarchical manner producing the inactive **glycogen synthase b**. Glycogen synthase is most active in its dephosphorylated form, known as **synthase a**.

Inactivation (phosphorylation) of glycogen synthase

Glycogen synthase has 737 amino acid residues and, of these, nine are serine residues that can be phosphorylated. Two of these are situated in the N-terminal region of the molecule (N-7 and N-10) and seven are located in the C-terminal region (C-30, C-34, C-38, C-42, C-46, C-87 and C-100). It has been demonstrated *in vitro* that at least seven protein kinases can phosphorylate glycogen synthase; five important examples are:

1 **Protein kinase A**, which phosphorylates sites C-87, C-100 and N-7.
2 **Glycogen synthase kinase-3 (GSK-3)**, which phosphorylates the cluster of serine residues at C-30, C-34, C-38 and C-42 (but not C-46). It is thought that GSK-3 plays a major role in insulin-stimulated glycogen synthesis as follows: during fasting, in the absence of insulin, GSK-3 is **constitutively active** and it phosphorylates glycogen synthase rendering it inactive. However, after feeding, insulin is present and causes the inactivation of GSK-3. This permits dephosphorylation and activation of glycogen synthase (Chapter 50).
3 **Phosphorylase kinase**, which phosphorylates the serine residue at N-7.
4 **Casein kinase-1**, which phosphorylates at N-10.
5 **Casein kinase-2**, which phosphorylates at C-46.

Activation (dephosphorylation) of glycogen synthase by protein phosphatase-1 (PP-1)

Protein phosphatase-1 dephosphorylates synthase b to produce **active glycogen synthase a**. Protein phosphatase-1 in turn is activated by insulin-generated signals mediated via PI-3 kinase (Chapter 50). This results in **phosphorylation** of site 1 of the glycogen-bound regulatory subunit G, thereby activating PP-1. Alternatively, **dephosphorylation** of site 2 of the regulatory subunit by protein phosphatase-2A allows reassociation of the catalytic and regulatory subunits to form active PP-1.

Role of glucose in the inhibition of phosphorylase in liver

Glucose, when abundant, is the major inhibitor of phosphorylase activity in liver. When glucose is bound to phosphorylase a, the latter acts as a better substrate for PP-1.

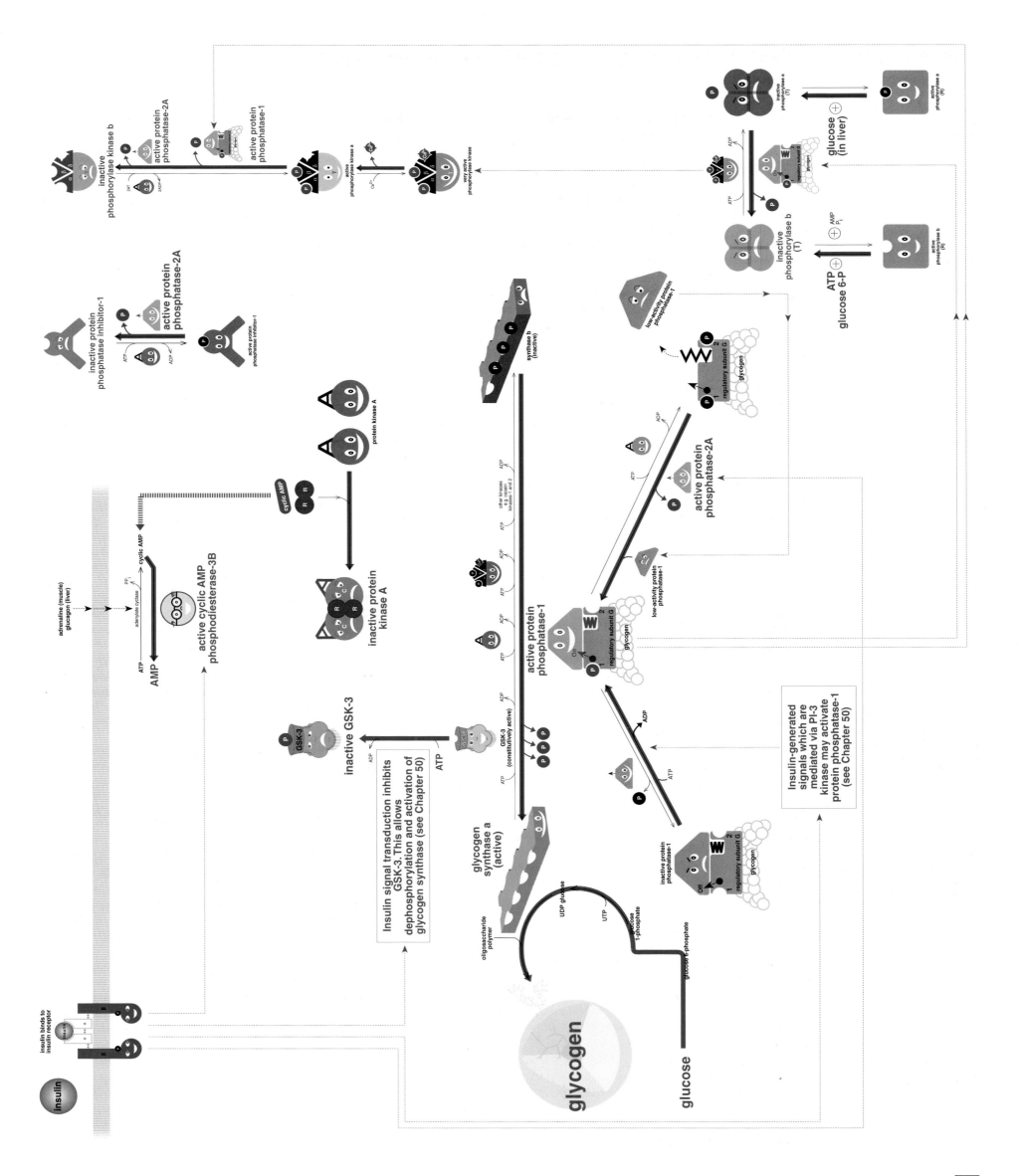

Regulation of glycolysis: overview exemplified by glycolysis in cardiac muscle

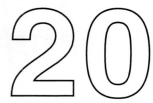

The regulatory mechanisms for glycolysis in cardiac muscle, skeletal muscle and liver are different.

The glycolytic pathway is ubiquitous but its physiological functions vary between different cell types. For example, whereas glycolysis can be very important for energy metabolism in cardiac and skeletal muscle, glucose is not a major source of energy for the liver. On the contrary, liver in the fed state tends to convert glucose to the fuel reserves glycogen and triacylglycerols. Indeed, apart from during the phase of food absorption in the fed state, the liver is usually not in glycolytic (i.e. glucose-**consuming**) mode, but instead **produces** glucose by either glycogenolysis or gluconeogenesis. Accordingly, regulation of glycolysis in **liver** is described in Chapters 21 & 23, while glycolysis in **skeletal muscle** is outlined in Chapter 22. Meanwhile, a general description of glycolysis is given below, while the chart opposite emphasizes the regulation in **cardiac muscle**.

Chart 20.1: The regulatory stages in glycolysis
Transport of glucose into the cell
Glucose in the surrounding fluid must cross the plasma membrane into the cell. This occurs by facilitated diffusion mediated by a family of proteins known as **glucose transporters (GLUT)**, which are distributed in different types of cells. **Muscle cells** and **adipocytes**, which are sensitive to insulin, have a transporter known as GLUT4. In response to insulin these are recruited from vesicles within the cell to the plasma membrane, where they increase glucose uptake (see Chapters 5 & 50). It should be noted that the transporters in **liver**, GLUT2 and in **red blood cells**, GLUT4, are constitutively located in the plasma membrane and so do not need insulin to be active.

Phosphorylation of glucose by hexokinase and glucokinase
Phosphorylation of glucose to glucose 6-phosphate in the **liver** (Chapters 21 & 23) is catalysed by the glucose-phosphorylating isoenzyme **glucokinase**, whereas in **muscle** the isoenzyme is **hexokinase**. Glucokinase (also known as hexokinase 4) is found only in **liver** and the **β-cells of the pancreas**, whereas hexokinase is widely distributed. The major difference between the isoenzymes is in their affinity for glucose. For glucokinase, the $K_{0.5}$ (glucose) is 10 mmol/l, whereas hexokinase has a K_m for glucose of 0.1 mmol/l. Thus the **liver** isoenzyme glucokinase is well adapted to cope with the high concentration surges of glucose in the blood during feeding. It should be remembered that dietary glucose from the intestines is absorbed into the hepatic portal vein, which transports the glucose directly to the liver at concentrations that can exceed 15 mmol/l. On the other hand, the high affinity of hexokinase for glucose ensures that, even if the intracellular concentration of glucose in **muscle** should fall as low as 0.1 mmol/l during a burst of strenuous exercise, the hexokinase reaction can still proceed at half its maximum velocity.

Another difference between hexokinase and glucokinase is that the former is inhibited by its product, **glucose 6-phosphate**, whereas glucokinase is not inhibited in this way. This ensures that, when the **liver** is presented with a large load of glucose after feeding it can be phosphorylated to glucose 6-phosphate prior to glycogenesis or lipogenesis. On the other hand, if glucose 6-phosphate accumulates in **muscle**, it inhibits hexokinase, decreases the glycolytic flux and thereby conserves glucose.

Glucokinase regulatory protein
It has been shown in **liver** that glucokinase is inactivated by sequestration with the **glucokinase regulatory protein (GKRP)**, which is bound within the hepatocyte nucleus. Very low concentrations of fructose liberate glucokinase from its regulatory protein and the active glucokinase molecule is translocated into the cytosol. This dramatic and novel control mechanism is described in Chapter 48.

Phosphofructokinase-1
Phosphofructokinase-1 (PFK-1) must be distinguished from phosphofructokinase-2 (PFK-2). PFK-2 produces **fructose-2,6 bisphosphate (F 2,6-bisP)**, which is a potent allosteric stimulator of PFK-1 (see below).

ATP, although a substrate for PFK-1, is also an allosteric inhibitor when present in increased concentrations, for example in the fed state. This inhibition by ATP is potentiated by **citrate** (see Chapter 11). However, this inhibition can be overcome by fructose 2,6-bisphosphate (see below).

Fructose 2,6-bisphosphate (F 2,6-bisP) is an important allosteric stimulator of glycolysis in muscle and inhibitor of gluconeogenesis in liver
Since F 2,6-bisP stimulates PFK-1, it has an important stimulatory effect on glycolysis. Furthermore, **in liver**, it stimulates PFK-1 (glycolysis) but **inhibits** fructose 1,6-bisphosphatase thereby decreasing gluconeogenesis (Chapters 21 & 23). The concentration of F 2,6-bisP **in liver** is down-regulated by glucagon, is upregulated in **cardiac muscle** by adrenaline, and in **skeletal muscle** is simply regulated by the concentration of fructose 6-phosphate. In liver and cardiac muscle, the hormones stimulate the production of cyclic AMP, which frees the active catalytic monomers of **protein kinase A (PKA)** (see Chapter 18), which in turn phosphorylates the 'bifunctional enzyme' phosphofructokinase-2/fructose 2,6-bisphosphatase (PFK-2/F 2,6-bisPase). Following phosphorylation, **in cardiac muscle**, PFK-2 is active and F 2,6-bisPase is inactive. This causes an increase in the concentration of F 2,6-bisP, which stimulates PFK-1, thereby increasing the rate of glycolysis.

The bifunctional enzyme, phosphofructokinase-2/fructose 2,6-bisphosphatase (PFK-2/F 2,6-bisPase)
The isoenzymes of PFK-2/F 2,6-bisPase found in cardiac muscle, liver and skeletal muscle are represented in Diagrams 20.1–20.3. The **cardiac isoenzyme** consists of 530 amino acids with a phosphorylation site at serine 466. Adrenaline through PKA phosphorylates this site and activates PFK-2, which favours the production of F 2,6-bisP, which stimulates PFK-1 and thus increases glycolysis (Chart 20.1).

The **liver isoenzyme** comprises 470 amino acids with a regulatory site at serine 32. Glucagon through PKA phosphorylates the bifunctional enzyme and **inactivates PFK-2** and **activates F 2,6-bisPase**. Thus in summary, **in liver** during fasting, glucagon causes concentrations of **F 2,6-bisP** to be decreased; **thus PFK-1** activity is **decreased**, the inhibition of F 1,6-bisPase by F 2,6-bisP is relieved, and so gluconeogenesis is stimulated (see Chapter 23). On the other hand, in the fed state when the insulin/glucagon ratio is high, dephosphorylation of PFK-2/F 2,6-bisPase occurs, PFK-2 is active, and F 2,6-bisP is formed, which stimulates PFK-1 and therefore glycolysis, providing pyruvate for fatty acid synthesis (see Chapter 21).

The **skeletal muscle** isoenzyme is the poor relation of the trio. It consists of only 450 amino acids and has no phosphorylation sites at either serine 32 or serine 466. Instead it is regulated simply by the availability of fructose 6-phosphate (F 6-P). When F 6-P is abundant, PFK-2 is active, **F 2,6-bisP** is formed, PFK-1 is stimulated and glycolysis is increased (see Chapter 22).

Pyruvate kinase
The inhibitory effects of alanine (allosteric) and glucagon (cyclic AMP/PKA-mediated phosphorylation) on the **liver isoenzyme** of pyruvate kinase are mainly concerned with directing the glycolytic pathway to the gluconeogenic mode. **NB:** The **muscle isoenzyme** of pyruvate kinase is not inhibited by alanine and so pyruvate, and thus alanine, can be formed when the glucose alanine cycle is operating (see Chapter 36). Also, the **muscle** isoenzyme is not subject to regulation by phosphorylation.

Fructose 1,6-bisphosphate activates pyruvate kinase allosterically by feed-forward stimulation. This has obvious advantages for energy metabolism in exercising **muscle** by enhancing the glycolytic flux at the end of the pathway. In **liver**, this feed-forward stimulatory effect of fructose 1,6-bisphosphate can overcome the inhibitory effect of alanine on pyruvate kinase.

Reference
For a review of the PFK-2/F 2,6-bisPase bifunctional enzyme see:
El-Maghrabi R.M., Noto F., Wu N. & Manes N. 6-phosphofructo-2-kinase/fructose-2,6-bisphosphatase: suiting structure to need, in a family of tissue-specific enzymes (2001) *Curr Opin Clin Nutr Metab Care*, **4**, 411–418.

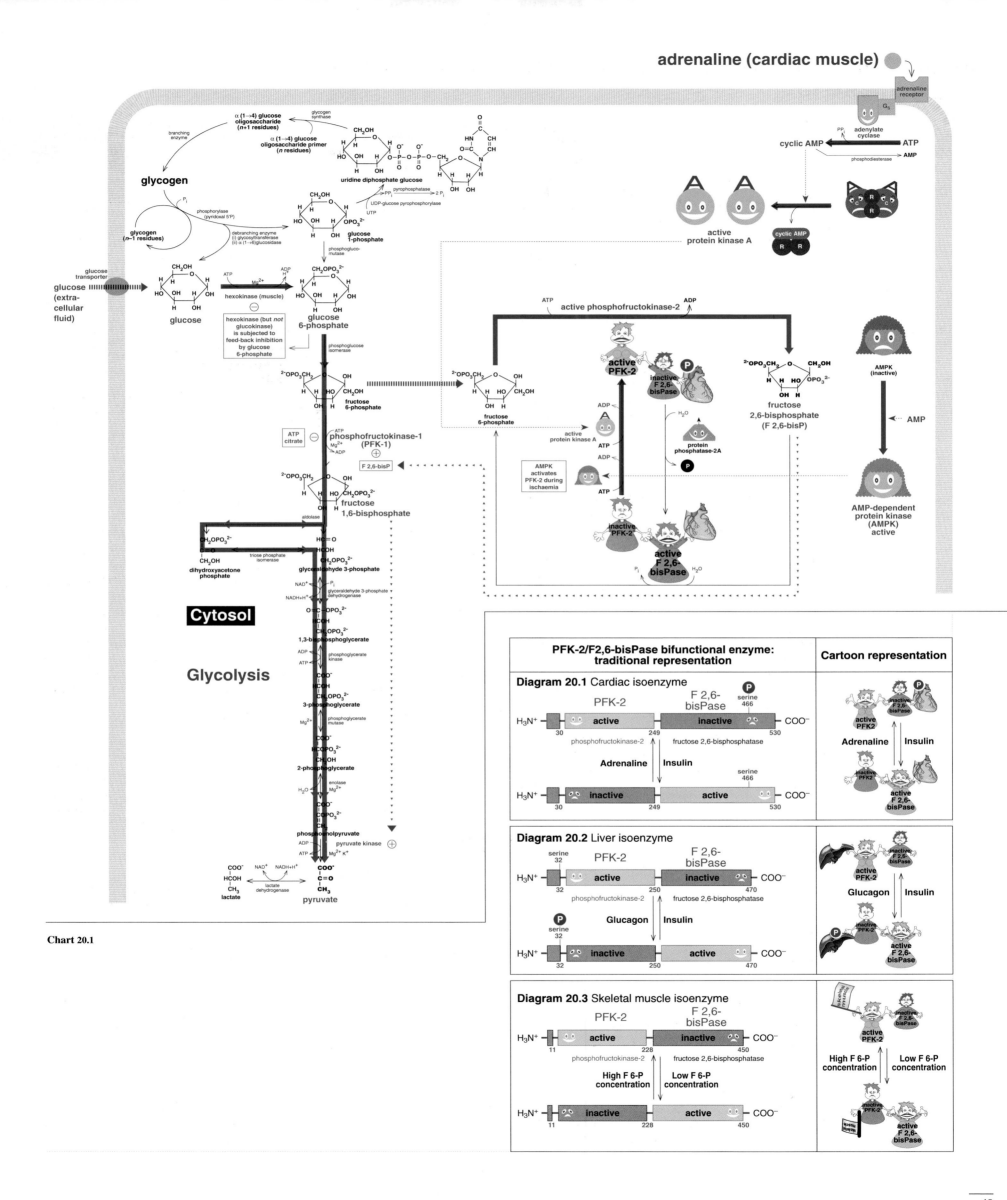

adrenaline (cardiac muscle)

glycogen

Cytosol

Glycolysis

Chart 20.1

**PFK-2/F2,6-bisPase bifunctional enzyme:
traditional representation** | **Cartoon representation**

Diagram 20.1 Cardiac isoenzyme

Diagram 20.2 Liver isoenzyme

Diagram 20.3 Skeletal muscle isoenzyme

Glycolysis and the pentose phosphate pathway collaborate in liver to make fat

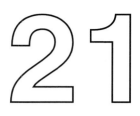

Chart 21.1 (opposite)
Metabolism of glucose to fat.

Liver is the biochemical factory of the body

The liver is the great provider and protector and, in metabolic terms, is like Mum, Dad and grandparents rolled up as one. Its extensive functions include an important role in glucose homeostasis during feeding and fasting. For example, after a meal when abundant glucose is delivered to the liver via the hepatic portal vein, glucose is metabolized to glycogen and stored in the liver. Also, during this period of feasting, glucose is metabolized to triacylglycerols such as tripalmitin (see Chart 21.1 opposite), which are exported to adipose tissue as very low-density lipoproteins (VLDL) for storage until needed during fasting.

Glycolysis operates in partnership with the pentose phosphate pathway to produce precursors needed for fatty acid synthesis

Unlike most tissues, for example muscle and nervous tissue, the liver does not use glycolysis for energy metabolism but instead depends on β-oxidation of fatty acids to provide ATP for biosynthetic pathways such as gluconeogenesis and urea synthesis (see Chapter 49). Instead, in liver, glycolysis operates in partnership with the pentose phosphate pathway to produce pyruvate, which is oxidatively decarboxylated to acetyl CoA, which is the precursor for fatty acid synthesis. However, as we have seen earlier, when there is an abundance of glucose, **ATP and citrate concentrations are increased and these compounds restrict the glycolytic pathway at the phosphofructokinase-1 (PFK-1) stage** (see Chapter 11). This obstruction to glycolytic flow means that glucose 6-phosphate is shunted through the pentose phosphate pathway, where it forms glyceraldehyde 3-phosphate and fructose 6-phosphate. The fate of this fructose 6-phosphate is described in the section on phosphofructokinase-1 below.

Glucose transport into liver cells

Glucose transport both into (fed state) and out of (fasting) liver cells is facilitated by the transport protein GLUT2, which has a very high K_m for glucose of 20 mmol/l. **Fanconi–Bickel syndrome** is a rare type of glycogen storage disease (type XI) caused by abnormal GLUT2 expressed in liver, intestinal, renal tubular cells, and pancreatic β-cells. Because of the in-out blockade of glucose transport, patients suffer **hepatorenal glycogen** accumulation and **fasting hypoglycaemia**, while after feeding they experience **transient hyperglycaemia**.

Glucokinase

As mentioned in Chapter 20, **in liver** glucose is phosphorylated to glucose 6-phosphate by **glucokinase**. This enzyme has a $K_{0.5}$ for glucose of 10 mmol/l. In other words it has a low affinity for glucose and is designed to cope with the enormous surges (≈15 mmol/l) of glucose arriving in the liver via the hepatic portal vein after feeding. The glucose 6-phosphate so formed can now make glycogen (Chapters 7 & 16). However, once the liver's glycogen stores are replete, glucose 6-phosphate is metabolized via **the pentose phosphate pathway** (see below).

Recently, it has been shown in liver that glucokinase is inactivated by sequestration with the glucokinase regulatory protein (GKRP), which is bound within the hepatocyte nucleus. Fructose 1-phosphate or high post-prandial concentrations of glucose liberate glucokinase from its regulatory protein and the active glucokinase is translocated into the cytosol. This dramatic and novel control mechanism is described in Chapter 48.

The pentose phosphate pathway

The pentose phosphate pathway plays an important role in liver, especially by providing reducing power in the form of NADPH. The formation of triacylglycerols needs a supply of reducing power in the form of NADPH (see Chart 21.1 opposite) as does the biosynthesis of cholesterol (Chapter 32). Also, NADPH is needed for the liver to maintain a supply of reduced glutathione as a defence against oxidative damage (Chapter 12).

The stoichiometry of the pentose phosphate pathway is best considered by following the fate of 3 glucose molecules as shown in Chart 21.1 opposite. The three molecules of glucose are phosphorylated by glucokinase to glucose 6-phosphate, which is oxidized by glucose 6-phosphate dehydrogenase to form 3 NADPH and 6-phosphogluconate. This is then oxidized and decarboxylated by 6-phosphogluconate dehydrogenase to form three more NADPH and ribulose 5-phosphate, and three carbons are lost as CO_2. The ribulose 5-phosphate is further metabolized by a series of reactions until the final products are glyceraldehyde 3-phosphate and two molecules of fructose 6-phosphate.

So the products of the pentose phosphate pathway are glyceraldehyde 3-phosphate and fructose 6-phosphate. Well clearly, there is no difficulty in the former being metabolized through glycolysis to pyruvate. However, the reader may be puzzled that fructose 6-phosphate is **upstream** of PFK-1 (which is inhibited by ATP and citrate (see Chapter 11)) and thus apparently incapable of further metabolism by glycolysis. The answer to this enigma depends on the regulation of PFK-1, which is explained below.

Phosphofructokinase-1 (PFK-1)

As explained above, the problem is that ATP and citrate inhibit PFK-1, and the fructose 6-phosphate formed by the pentose phosphate pathway is upstream of this blockade. The question is how can this fructose 6-phosphate be metabolized by glycolysis to pyruvate and onwards to fatty acids? The answer to this predicament is **fructose 2,6-bisphosphate (F 2,6-bisP)**, which is produced by the liver isoenzyme of the bifunctional phosphofructokinase-2/fructose 2,6-bisphosphatase (PFK-2/F 2,6-bisPase) described in Chapter 20. F 2,6-bisP is a potent allosteric stimulator of PFK-1 and so it overcomes the inhibition caused by ATP and citrate. The regulation of PFK-2/F 2,6-bisPase is described below.

Finally, there is recent evidence that **ribose 1,5-bisphosphate** (formed from ribulose 5-phosphate in the cooperative pentose phosphate pathway) stimulates PFK-1 and inhibits its opposing enzyme, fructose 1,6-bisphosphatase.

Phosphofructokinase-2/fructose 2,6-bisphosphatase (PFK-2/F 2,6-bisPase)

After feeding, when insulin concentrations are raised, the bifunctional PFK-2/F 2,6-bisPase is dephosphorylated by protein phosphatase 2A. This activates PFK-2 activity, which results in production of F 2,6-bisP, which stimulates PFK-1 and increases the rate of glycolysis as described above. There is evidence for further cooperation with the pentose phosphate pathway in that **xylulose 5-phosphate** enhances dephosphorylation of PFK-2/F 2,6-bisPase.

Pyruvate kinase (PK)

During feeding, pyruvate kinase (PK) is allosterically stimulated by fructose 1,6-bisphosphate in an example of feed-forward stimulation. This serves to overcome the allosteric inhibition of liver PK caused by alanine which occurs during fasting. Also, insulin activates protein phosphatase 2A, which dephosphorylates and activates liver PK reversing its phosphorylated inactive state that prevails during fasting.

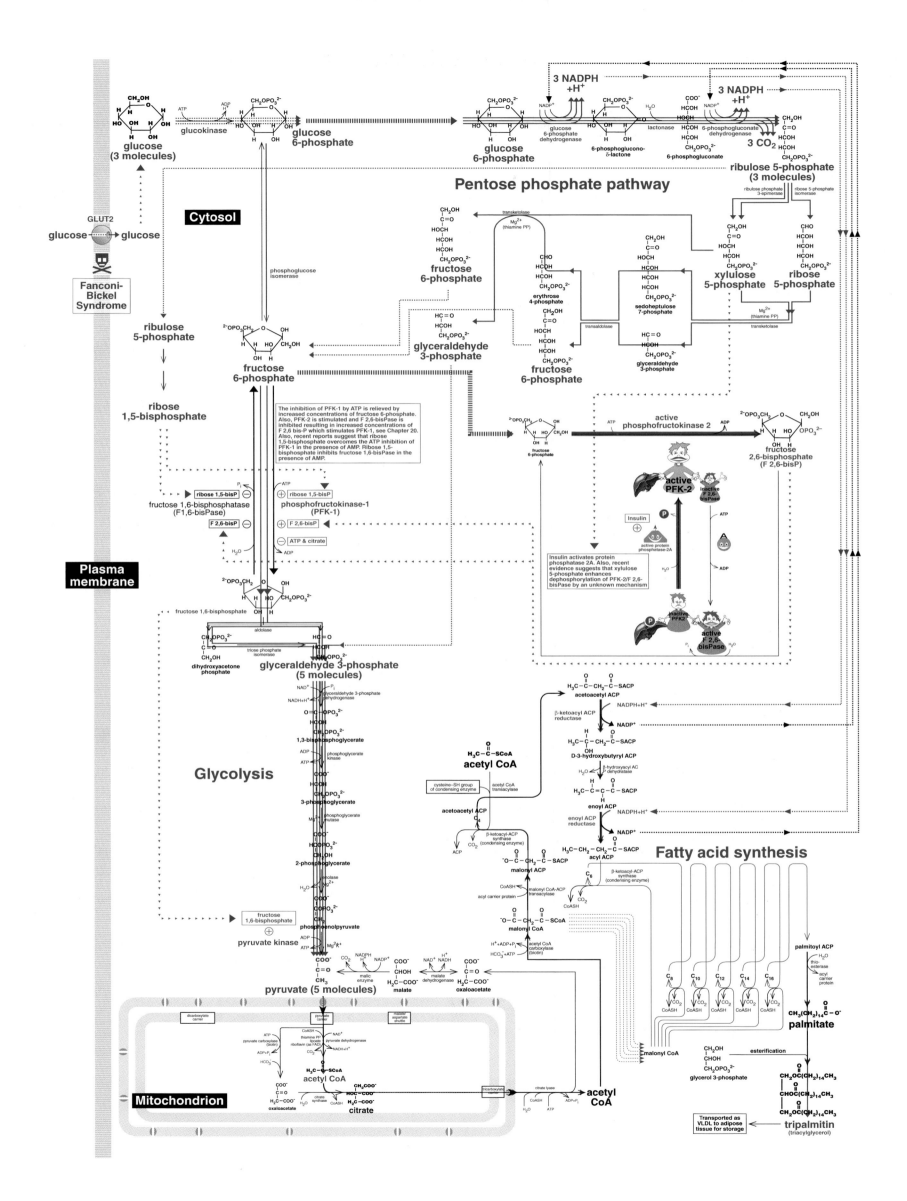

Glycolysis in skeletal muscle: biochemistry of sport and exercise

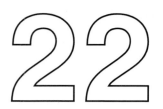

Chart 22.2 (opposite) Aerobic production of ATP for muscle contraction.

Chart 22.1 Anaerobic production of ATP for muscle contraction.

Anaerobic ATP production

The ATP used for contraction by the white, type II (fast-twitch) muscle fibres is provided anaerobically during explosive bursts of muscle activity, such as sprint races or other athletic events. In track events such as the 100 metres, ATP is provided both by the phosphagen **phosphocreatine** and a 1000-fold increase in glycolysis (see Chart 22.1). Phosphocreatine hydrolysis provides **inorganic phosphate (P_i)** for phosphorylase, which is activated by Ca^{2+} released from the sarcoplasmic reticulum, and also by adrenaline through the cyclic AMP signalling system (Chapter 18). Lactate and hydrogen ions are produced, with the latter being buffered by bicarbonate in the plasma to form carbonic acid and then carbon dioxide, which is expired from the lungs.

The AMP formed by **adenylate kinase** is deaminated to form inosine monophosphate (IMP), which is a potent stimulator of phosphorylase. It is also dephosphorylated by **5′-nucleotidase** producing **adenosine**, which binds to adenosine A_2-receptors on blood vessels causing vasodilation. Accordingly, adenosine has been described as a 'retaliatory metabolite' that retaliates against hypoxia in exercising muscle by increasing the supply of oxygen via the blood.

Aerobic ATP production
Glycogen and fatty acids are used as fuel

The ATP used for contraction by the red, type I (slow-twitch) muscle fibres is generated aerobically for endurance events such as the marathon (Chart 22.2). Glycogen and fatty acids are the principal fuels used. The latter originate from three possible sources. Most important are (i) fatty acids mobilized from adipose tissue by hormone-sensitive lipase and (ii) fatty acids from plasma VLDL mobilized by lipoprotein lipase; (iii) of lesser importance are fatty acids formed by hydrolysis of the intramuscular triacylglycerol.

Glycogen exhaustion causes the athlete to 'hit the wall'

Both fatty acids and glycogen form acetyl CoA, which is oxidized by Krebs cycle. ATP is generated by oxidative phosphorylation in the respiratory chain. The abundant supply of acetyl CoA condenses with a matching supply of oxaloacetate. Although this is regenerated by Krebs cycle (see Chapter 24), supplementary oxaloacetate is needed. The supply of this is maintained by **anaplerotic reactions**, notably the Krebs cycle intermediate **succinyl CoA** produced by catabolism of **isoleucine** and **valine**.

If muscle glycogen is exhausted, then fatty acids alone are used as fuel. However, their metabolism generates ATP at only half the rate compared with glycogen and so the long-distance runner is forced to slow down dramatically.

The sprint to the tape is fuelled by glycogen

The abundant acetyl CoA restricts the activity of pyruvate dehydrogenase. This limits glycolysis and helps to conserve glycogen throughout the race and, if reserves permit, enables a powerful **anaerobic** sprint to the finish.

The glucose transporters

The principal glucose transporter in skeletal muscle is GLUT4, which is recruited to the sarcolemma by insulin and also by exercise. The glucose transporter GLUT1 is probably more important for basal uptake of glucose into muscle cells, and for replenishing the glycogen reserves with glucose formed from lactate by the liver following recovery from exercise.

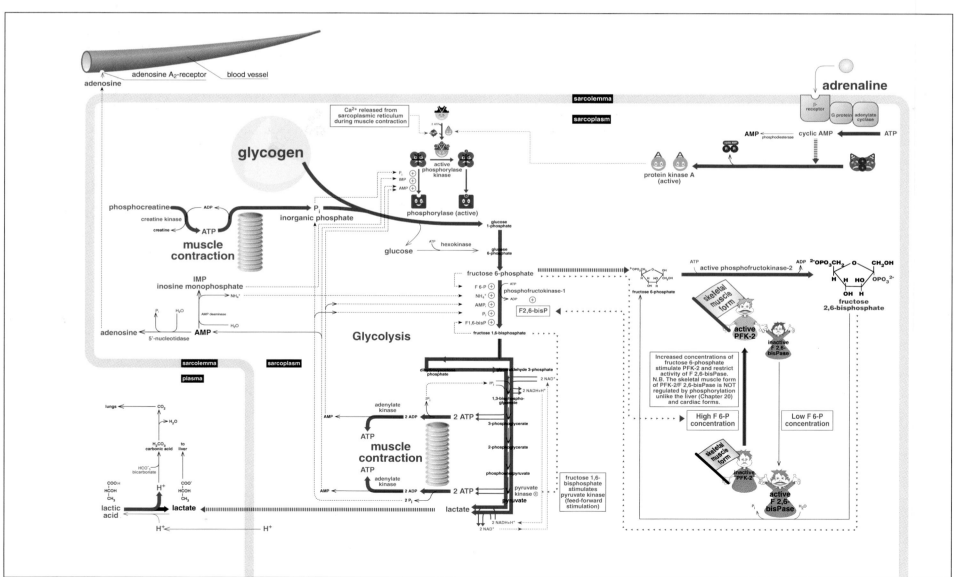

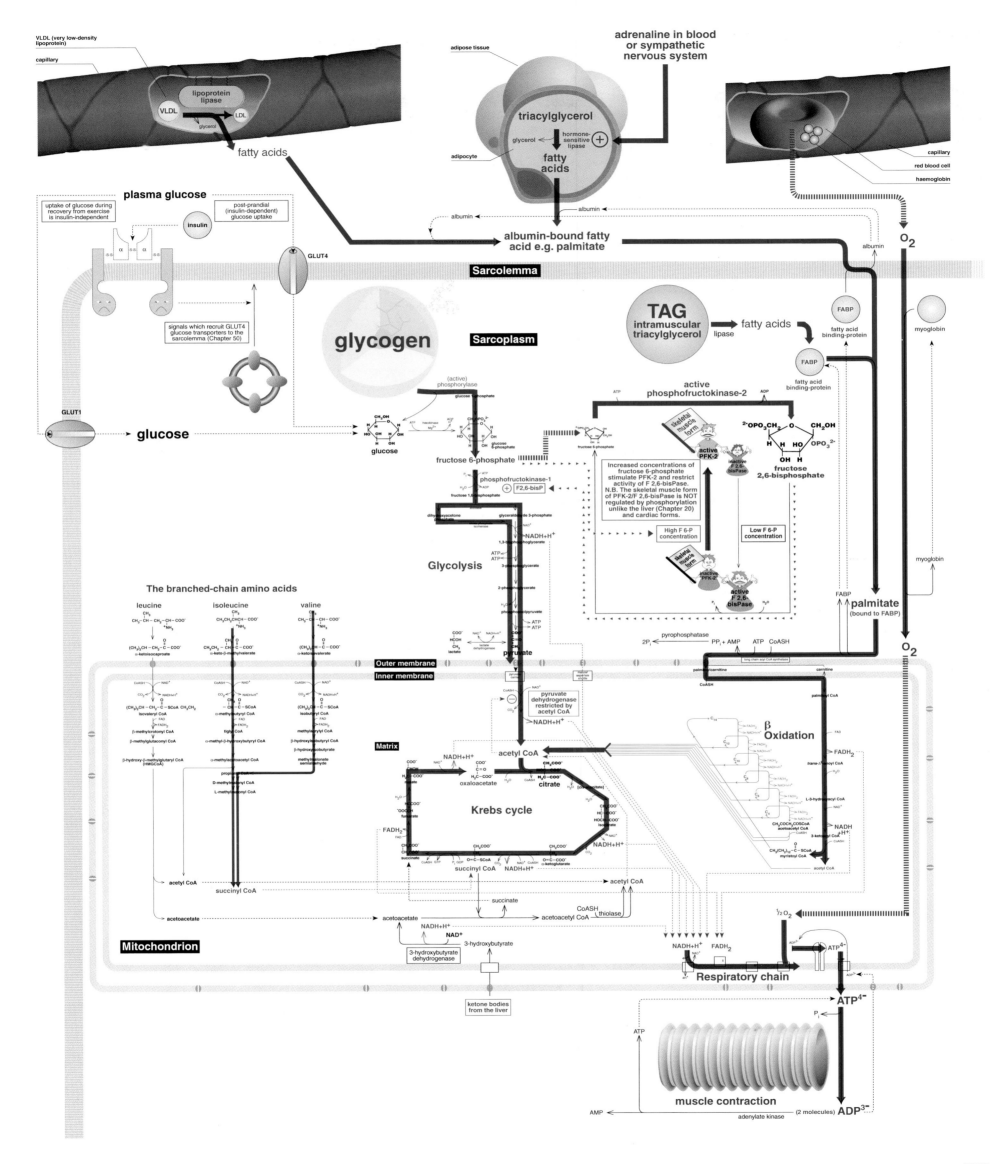

Regulation of gluconeogenesis

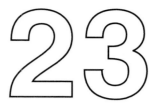

Gluconeogenesis maintains the blood glucose concentration during fasting and starvation

The body's first and foremost reserve for maintaining the blood glucose concentration during fasting is liver glycogen. However, once this reserve is exhausted, glucose must be made from non-carbohydrate precursors. We have seen that the most abundant fuel reserve, the fatty acids in triacylglycerol, cannot be converted to glucose by mammals (see Chapter 14). However, glucose can be made from glycerol and lactate, and from amino acids formed by proteolysis of muscle proteins (see Chapters 8 & 36). This process is known as gluconeogenesis. It occurs mainly in the liver but, during prolonged starvation, it is also active in kidney cortex.

Chart 23.1: Regulation of gluconeogenesis
Dependency of gluconeogenesis on the oxidation of fatty acids

Gluconeogenesis, which operates during starvation, is linked to the mobilization of fat and the oxidation of fatty acids e.g. **palmitate** in the mitochondrion. The latter results in the formation of large amounts of acetyl CoA, NADH and ATP, with the following effects on mitochondrial reactions:

1 **Isocitrate dehydrogenase** is inhibited by NADH.
2 **Pyruvate dehydrogenase** is inhibited by acetyl CoA, ATP and NADH.
3 **Pyruvate carboxylase** is stimulated by acetyl CoA.
4 The equilibrium of the mitochondrial **malate dehydrogenase** reaction is displaced to favour the reduction of oxaloacetate to malate.
5 ATP (and GTP via the nucleoside diphosphate kinase reaction) from the β-oxidation and respiratory chain pathways is used as a co-substrate for the pyruvate carboxylase, phosphoenolpyruvate carboxykinase and phosphoglycerate kinase reactions.

Gluconeogenic precursors

Amino acids, particularly **alanine**, are important gluconeogenic precursors, but they must first be metabolized to cytosolic oxaloacetate (see Chapter 38). **Glycerol**, derived from triacylglycerols in white adipose tissue, is also an important gluconeogenic precursor. It is phosphorylated in the liver by **glycerol kinase** to form glycerol 3-phosphate, which in turn is oxidized by glycerol 3-phosphate dehydrogenase to form the gluconeogenic intermediate **dihydroxyacetone phosphate**. Finally, **lactate**, produced for example by anaerobic glycolysis in red blood cells or muscle, is also used for gluconeogenesis.

Hormonal regulation of gluconeogenesis

Glucagon is an important hormone in the early fasting state. It stimulates **hormone-sensitive lipase** through the action of protein kinase A.

Furthermore, it inhibits pyruvate kinase by the same mechanism thereby restricting glycolysis. Glucagon also has effects on the synthesis of certain enzymes. It increases synthesis of the aminotransferases, phosphoenolpyruvate carboxykinase and glucose 6-phosphatase, which favour gluconeogenesis.

Regulatory enzymes
Pyruvate carboxylase

Pyruvate carboxylase, which converts pyruvate to oxaloacetate, is stimulated by acetyl CoA. **NB:** Pyruvate dehydrogenase, which competes for pyruvate as a substrate, is inactivated by acetyl CoA.

Phosphoenolpyruvate carboxykinase (PEPCK)

PEPCK decarboxylates oxaloacetate to phosphoenolpyruvate (PEP). It requires GTP, which can be obtained from ATP by the nucleoside diphosphate kinase reaction. PEPCK activity is induced in the long term when the ratio of glucagon to insulin is high.

In theory, PEP could be converted to pyruvate, enter Krebs cycle as oxaloacetate and be reconverted to PEP in a futile cycle. This does not happen, because liver pyruvate kinase is inactivated by protein kinase A (due to the presence of glucagon), and is inhibited by alanine, which is present in increased concentrations during gluconeogenic conditions (see Chapter 36).

Fructose 1,6-bisphosphatase (F 1,6-bisPase)

Regulation of this enzyme has been mentioned in Chapter 20. **F 1,6-bisPase is inhibited by fructose 2,6-bisphosphate (F 2,6-bisP)**. Glucagon, which is secreted by the α-cells of the pancreas in response to a low blood glucose concentration, stimulates the breakdown of F 2,6-bisP in liver through the action of protein kinase A on fructose 2,6-bisphosphatase (F 2,6-bisPase) activity (see Chapter 20). Removal of the allosteric inhibitor F 2,6-bisP results in an increase in F 1,6-bisPase activity. The decrease in F 2,6-bisP also results in reduced PFK-1 activity and a further reduction in glycolysis. Fructose 1,6-bisPase deficiency is described in Chapter 48.

Glucose 6-phosphatase

Glucose 6-phosphatase is located on the luminal surface of the endoplasmic reticulum in liver cells (see Diagram 23.1). Its substrate, glucose 6-phosphate, is transported by a translocator from the cytosol into the lumen of the endoplasmic reticulum, where it is hydrolysed to glucose and inorganic phosphate (P_i). The reaction products are then transported into the cytosol by a glucose translocator GLUT7 and an inorganic phosphate (P_i) translocator. Glycogen storage disease Type I is due to deficiency of glucose 6-phosphatase activity (see Chapter 16).

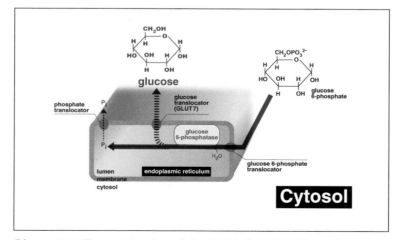

Diagram 23.1 Glucose 6-phosphatase is localized on the inside of the rough endoplasmic reticulum membrane. **NB :** The ribosomes are not shown.

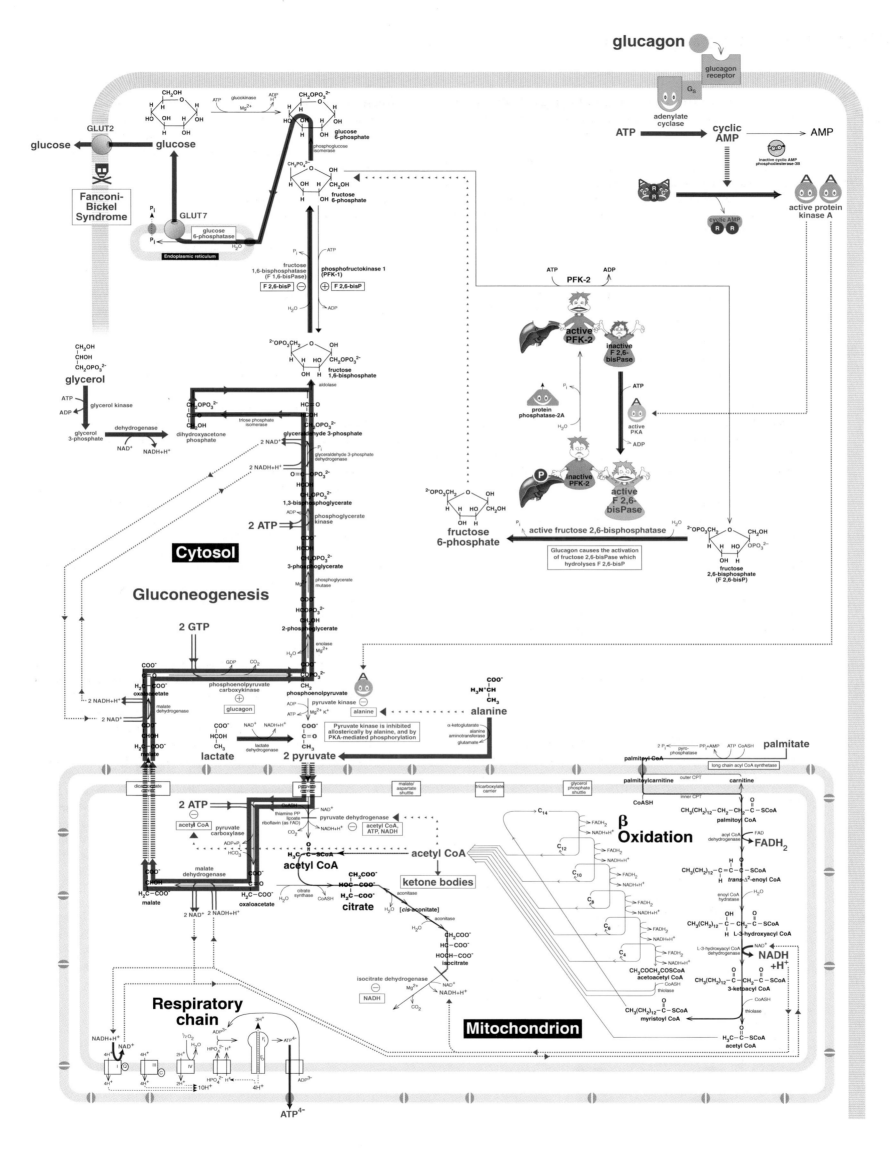

Chart 23.1
Regulation of gluconeogenesis.

Regulation of Krebs cycle

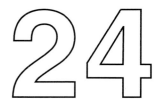

Krebs cycle – the central junction of metabolism

Krebs cycle is found in nearly all mammalian cells, with the notable exception of mature red blood cells, which lack mitochondria. The cycle oxidizes acetyl CoA derived from carbohydrates, ketone bodies, fatty acids and amino acids, to produce NADH and $FADH_2$ for ATP synthesis in the respiratory chain. Furthermore, components of the cycle form essential links with the pathways for gluconeogenesis, lipogenesis and amino acid metabolism. As such, regulation of Krebs cycle must satisfy the diverse metabolic demands of these pathways in the various tissues with their different functions. For example, glucose is a premium fuel because of its vital role as a respiratory substrate for the brain and red blood cells. Because the body has a limited capacity to store carbohydrate, it must be conserved and not exhausted in a frenzied fit of exercise by the fuel-guzzling muscles, which can very happily use fatty acids as an alternative energy source. Pyruvate dehydrogenase (PDH) can therefore be thought of as the 'Minister for Glucose Conservation' since it determines whether or not pyruvate (which is mainly derived from carbohydrate or amino acids) enters Krebs cycle for oxidation.

The activity of Krebs cycle is controlled by the regulation of pyruvate dehydrogenase and isocitrate dehydrogenase.

Regulation of the pyruvate dehydrogenase (PDH) complex

Pyruvate dehydrogenase, although not a component of Krebs cycle, has a commanding role in regulating the flux of glycolytic metabolites into the cycle. It is a multienzyme complex consisting of three component enzymes. These enzymes (E_1, pyruvate dehydrogenase; E_2, acetyl transferase; and E_3, dihydrolipoyl dehydrogenase) are responsible for decarboxylating the pyruvate, transferring the acetyl residue to CoA to form acetyl CoA, and oxidatively regenerating the intermediary lipoate involved. Associated with the complex are two enzymes that have regulatory roles (see Diagram 24.1). One, PDH kinase, is a protein kinase that is specific for PDH. Its role is to phosphorylate and thus inactivate the pyruvate dehydrogenase component of the complex. The other, PDH phosphatase, is a specific PDH phosphatase that overcomes this inhibition by removing the phosphate groups, thereby activating PDH. PDH is also regulated by the availability of its coenzymes NAD^+ and CoA; i.e. its activity is decreased when high ratios of $NADH/NAD^+$ and acetyl CoA/CoA prevail.

Diagram 24.1: Regulation of PDH by phosphorylation and dephosphorylation

When the energy charge of the cell is high, i.e. the ratio of ATP to ADP is increased, PDH kinase is active. E_1 is therefore phosphorylated at three sites and its activity is inhibited. Conversely, PDH kinase is inhibited by pyruvate, and this leads to activation of PDH in the presence of its substrate.

In muscle, PDH phosphatase is activated during muscle contraction, when cytosolic and mitochondrial concentrations of calcium ions are increased. In adipose tissue, PDH phosphatase is activated by insulin. In both of these cases, dephosphorylation of PDH occurs and PDH activity is stimulated.

Isocitrate dehydrogenase (ICDH)

ICDH is inhibited by the high ratio of $NADH/NAD^+$ that prevails in the high-energy state. When ICDH is inhibited, flux through this section of Krebs cycle is restricted.

The purine nucleotide cycle

When large quantities of acetyl CoA are available for oxidation by Krebs cycle, the availability of oxaloacetate for the citrate synthase reaction may become a rate-limiting factor. It is known that the purine nucleotide cycle, first described by Lowenstein, is very active in muscle during exercise (see Chart 24.1). This cycle generates **fumarate** from **aspartate** in the presence of **GTP** in circumstances when the AMP concentration is increased (e.g. when the ATP concentration is decreased, as during muscle contraction). The purine nucleotide cycle thus via fumarate provides an **anaplerotic** (i.e. 'topping up') supply of mitochondrial **malate** to produce **oxaloacetate** in an effort to match the abundant supply of acetyl CoA presented for oxidation by Krebs cycle.

As would be expected, patients with **muscle AMP deaminase deficiency** (myoadenylate deaminase deficiency) suffer cramps and myalgias, and fatigue easily after exercise. AMP deaminase activity in the other tissues of these patients is normal.

The glucose-fatty acid cycle

This was described in 1963 by Randle, Garland, Hales and Newsholme. However, it is not a cycle of intermediary metabolites like Krebs cycle but it shows that **the relationship between glucose and fatty acids is integrated and reciprocal**. It explains that if muscle has a choice between glucose and fatty acids as fuel, **muscle prefers fatty acids** and mechanisms exist to restrict glucose metabolism. This is because β-oxidation of fatty acids increases the concentration ratios of acetyl CoA/CoA, $NADH/NAD^+$ and ATP/ADP, which inhibits PDH (see Chart 24.1 and Diagram 24.1) and prevents the oxidation of pyruvate (from glycolysis) thus conserving glucose. This is especially important during starvation. However, a disadvantage is that after feeding when there is an abundance of both glucose and fatty acids, this process reduces the uptake of glucose by muscle and contributes to insulin resistance, see Chapters 53 and 54.

Reference

Randle P.J., Garland P.B., Hales C.N. & Newsholme E.A. (1963) The glucose-fatty acid cycle: its role in insulin sensitivity and the metabolic disturbances of diabetes mellitus. *Lancet* (**i**), 785–89.

Diagram 24.1 Regulation of pyruvate dehydrogenase by phosphorylation and dephosphorylation.

Debating forum. Krebs cycle: is it time to change the name of the bedrock of metabolism?

Now call me a pedant if you will, but I feel the time has come to consider the nomenclature which can confuse understanding of metabolism. Professor Sir Hans Krebs was the principal contributor to the discovery of two metabolic cycles: the Krebs Henseleit cycle (1923) popularly known as the urea cycle or ornithine cycle; and the Krebs cycle (1937), otherwise known as the tricarboxylic acid (TCA) cycle, or citric acid cycle. Strictly speaking, it is ambiguous to refer to these pathways simply as Krebs cycle since this could mean either the former or the latter. Moreover, the term 'tricarboxylic acid cycle' implies that tricarboxylic acids are cycled which, of course, they are not; it is oxaloacetate (the base of a dicarboxylic acid) which condenses with acetyl CoA and which is recycled following the oxidation of the acetyl CoA. Similarly, 'citric acid cycle' is misleading since citric acid, or more importantly at physiological pH its base citrate, is an intermediate and is not recycled.

The intermediate which **is recycled** as mentioned above is **oxaloacetate**. The reader should be aware of this and should think of this pathway as '*the Krebs **oxaloacetate** cycle for the oxidation of acetyl CoA*'. In the meantime, until an international nomenclature committee adopts (or ignores) this proposal, the reader should use any of the unsatisfactory names in common use, although this author prefers 'Krebs cycle'.

Likewise, the commonly used term 'urea cycle' is misleading since it is **ornithine** which is recycled in the more accurately described 'Krebs Henseleit **ornithine cycle** for the production of urea'. In practice, the succinct term 'urea cycle' is invariably used but this awaits a future campaign.

Chart 24.1
Regulation of Krebs cycle.

Regulation of fatty acid oxidation: mobilization of fatty acids from storage in adipose tissue

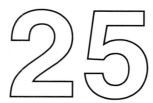

During exercise, periods of stress or starvation, the triacylglycerol reserves in adipose tissue are mobilized as fatty acids for oxidation as a respiratory fuel. This is analogous to the mobilization of glycogen as glucose units; it occurs under similar circumstances, and is under similar hormonal control.

Fatty acids are a very important energy substrate in red muscle. In liver they are metabolized to the ketone bodies. Because fatty acids are hydrophobic, they are transported in the blood bound to albumin. They can serve most cells as a respiratory fuel, with the notable exceptions of brain and red blood cells, which lack the enzymes for fatty acid oxidation.

Regulation of the utilization of fatty acids appears to be at four levels:

1 Lipolysis of triacylglycerol to form the free fatty acids.
2 Re-esterification of the fatty acids or, alternatively, their mobilization from adipose tissue.
3 Transport of the acyl CoA esters into the mitochondrion.
4 Availability of FAD and NAD⁺ for β-oxidation.

The first two of these will be considered now and the other two will be covered in Chapter 26.

Chart 25.1 (opposite) The triacylglycerol / fatty acid cycle.

Lipolysis in adipose tissue

Lipolysis in adipose tissue is controlled by **hormone-sensitive lipase (HSL)**. This enzyme hydrolyses triacylglycerol to monoacylglycerol, which in turn is hydrolysed by **monoacylglycerol lipase**. In Chart 25.1, for example, **tripalmitin** is converted to three molecules of **palmitate** and one molecule of **glycerol**.

Diagram 25.1 Mobilization of fatty acids in adipose tissue. The isoform of acetyl CoA carboxylase found in lipogenic tissue (adipose tissue, liver and mammary gland) is ACC-α. In skeletal muscle and heart, ACC-β is present.

Lipolysis is stimulated by **adrenaline** during exercise and by **noradrenaline** from noradrenergic nerves, and is inhibited by **insulin**. Curiously, although **glucagon** stimulates lipolysis *in vitro* it has no effect on human HSL *in vivo* (see Diagram 25.1). The mechanism involves protein kinase A, as described in Chapter 18, which stimulates HSL and inhibits acetyl CoA carboxylase-α by phosphorylating serine 77. Also, AMP-dependent protein kinase, which is activated when it senses the low energy state of the cell when ATP is hydrolysed to AMP, phosphorylates serine 79, 1200 and 1215. Furthermore, as a long-term adaptation to prolonged starvation, **cortisol** stimulates the synthesis of HSL, thereby increasing its concentration and activity. Conversely, in the fed state, HSL is inhibited by **insulin**.

Mobilization of fatty acids: the triacylglycerol–fatty acid cycle

We have seen how triacylglycerol is hydrolysed by HSL to **free fatty acids** and **glycerol**. *However, glycerol kinase is absent from white adipose tissue and so the glycerol cannot be metabolized further (the classical opinion, but see opposite!).* Instead, it goes to the liver where hepatic glycerol kinase forms glycerol 3-phosphate, which undergoes gluconeogenesis.

In adipose tissue, the **free fatty acids** liberated by lipolysis have two possible fates within the adipocyte:

1 They can be released from the adipocyte for β-oxidation elsewhere, for example, by muscle or liver.
2 Alternatively, they can be re-esterified with **glycerol 3-phosphate**. This is illustrated in Chart 25.1, which shows how fatty acids (e.g. palmitate) are activated by acyl CoA synthetase to form acyl CoA. This then combines first with **glycerol 3-phosphate** to form lysophosphatidate, then proceeds via other intermediates to form **triacylglycerol**.

The importance of **insulin** in maintaining this cycle should be noted. The GLUT4 glucose transporter in adipose tissue needs insulin to be effective, therefore during fasting the cycle is disrupted. As a result, glycerol 3-phosphate is not formed by glycolysis and so is not available for re-esterification of the fatty acids formed by HSL. Consequently, in the absence of insulin, these free fatty acids are released from the adipocyte for use as a respiratory fuel by the tissues.

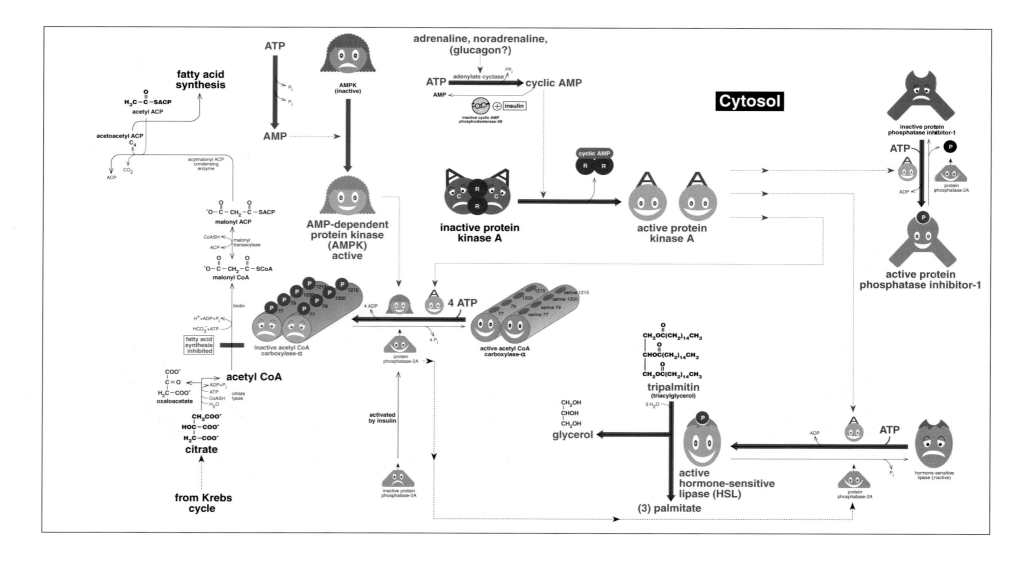

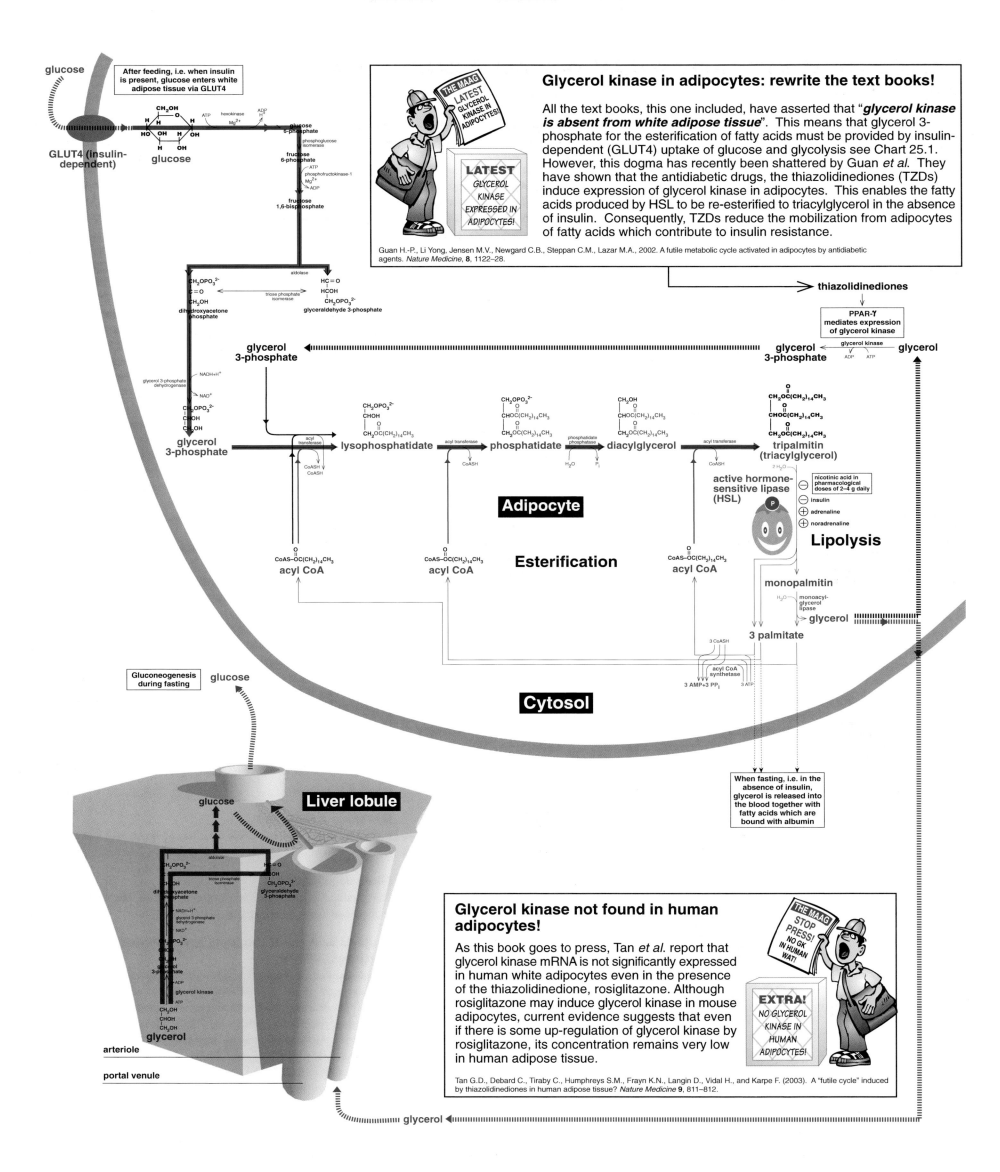

Glycerol kinase in adipocytes: rewrite the text books!

All the text books, this one included, have asserted that "**glycerol kinase is absent from white adipose tissue**". This means that glycerol 3-phosphate for the esterification of fatty acids must be provided by insulin-dependent (GLUT4) uptake of glucose and glycolysis see Chart 25.1. However, this dogma has recently been shattered by Guan *et al.* They have shown that the antidiabetic drugs, the thiazolidinediones (TZDs) induce expression of glycerol kinase in adipocytes. This enables the fatty acids produced by HSL to be re-esterified to triacylglycerol in the absence of insulin. Consequently, TZDs reduce the mobilization from adipocytes of fatty acids which contribute to insulin resistance.

Guan H.-P., Li Yong, Jensen M.V., Newgard C.B., Steppan C.M., Lazar M.A., 2002. A futile metabolic cycle activated in adipocytes by antidiabetic agents. *Nature Medicine*, **8**, 1122–28.

Glycerol kinase not found in human adipocytes!

As this book goes to press, Tan *et al.* report that glycerol kinase mRNA is not significantly expressed in human white adipocytes even in the presence of the thiazolidinedione, rosiglitazone. Although rosiglitazone may induce glycerol kinase in mouse adipocytes, current evidence suggests that even if there is some up-regulation of glycerol kinase by rosiglitazone, its concentration remains very low in human adipose tissue.

Tan G.D., Debard C., Tiraby C., Humphreys S.M., Frayn K.N., Langin D., Vidal H., and Karpe F. (2003). A "futile cycle" induced by thiazolidinediones in human adipose tissue? *Nature Medicine* **9**, 811–812.

Fatty acid oxidation and the carnitine shuttle

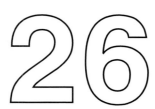

Chart 26.1 (opposite) The carnitine shuttle and the β-oxidation of fatty acids.

The release of fatty acids from triacylglycerols in adipose tissue is regulated by hormone-sensitive lipase (see Chapter 25). The fatty acids, bound to albumin, are then transported to the liver and muscles for utilization. The rate of uptake by these tissues of the fatty acids is proportional to the concentration of the latter in the blood. In all tissues, the rate of β-oxidation is regulated by the availability of coenzyme A, which is regenerated following utilization of acetyl CoA for ketogenesis in liver, and by citrate synthase in muscle. In liver, β-oxidation is regulated by controlling mitochondrial uptake of fatty acids by the carnitine shuttle. In muscle, an important regulatory factor is the availability of the coenzymes NAD$^+$ and FAD, which are regenerated from their reduced forms when ATP is produced by oxidative phosphorylation in exercising muscle.

Transport of activated fatty acids into the mitochondrial matrix by the carnitine shuttle is inhibited by malonyl CoA in liver

Fatty acids are activated by long-chain acyl CoA synthetase to form acyl CoA, for example **palmitoyl CoA** as shown in Chart 26.1. A transport system, **the carnitine shuttle**, is needed to enable long-chain fatty acids to cross the inner mitochondrial membrane. **In liver**, this transport is inhibited by **malonyl CoA** (and there is some evidence this may be significant in skeletal muscle and pancreatic β-cells). Since malonyl CoA is produced during fatty acid synthesis, this ensures that the newly formed fatty acids are not immediately transported into the mitochondrion for degradation by β-oxidation.

The carnitine shuttle consists of **carnitine/acylcarnitine translocase** and two **carnitine-palmitoyl transferases (CPT)**: an outer **CPT I** and an inner **CPT II**. Although not shown in the Chart, it is possible that *in vivo*, CPT II and membrane-bound very-long-chain acyl CoA dehydrogenase (VLCAD) are contiguous to facilitate substrate channelling.

Availability of the coenzymes FAD and NAD$^+$ for β-oxidation

The various acyl CoA dehydrogenases (see below) need a supply of FAD, which must be regenerated from FADH$_2$ by oxidation via the **electron-transfer flavoprotein (ETF)** and the respiratory chain. Likewise, the **3-hydroxyacyl CoA dehydrogenases** of β-oxidation require NAD$^+$ as coenzyme. However, they have to compete with the three NAD$^+$-dependent dehydrogenases of Krebs cycle for the limited NAD$^+$ available. In exercising muscle when both pathways are highly active, β-oxidation may be limited by the supply of NAD$^+$.

The acyl CoA dehydrogenases

Mitochondria contain four FAD-dependent, acyl CoA dehydrogenases, which act on very-long-, long-, medium- and short-chain fatty acids, although there is some overlap of specificities. Recently, it has been discovered that these are located in both the matrix and the inner membrane of the mitochondrion.

Very-long-chain acyl CoA dehydrogenase (VLCAD, active with C_{12}–C_{24} fatty acids) is situated in the inner membrane. It has an FAD prosthetic group, which is reduced to FADH$_2$ and the electrons transferred to another FAD prosthetic group of the **electron-transfer flavoprotein (ETF)**, which is a soluble matrix protein (see Chart 26.1). The electrons now pass to **ETF:ubiquinone oxidoreductase (ETF:QO)** – an iron-sulphur flavoprotein located in the inner membrane – before passing to ubiquinone (Q) and entering the respiratory chain. *NB: The carnitine shuttle is unable to transport **very-long-**chain fatty acids and so, confusingly, the principal substrates for VLCAD in mitochondria are **long**-chain fatty acids. Oxidation of very-long-chain fatty acids occurs in the peroxisomes (see Chapter 30).*

The other three acyl CoA dehydrogenases, which are located in the matrix, are: **long-chain acyl CoA dehydrogenase (LCAD**, C_8–C_{20}), **medium-chain acyl CoA dehydrogenase (MCAD**, C_4–C_{12}), and **short-chain acyl CoA dehydrogenase (SCAD**, C_4 and C_6). **NB:** In humans the function of LCAD is not understood and so it has not been shown in Chart 26.1 opposite.

Δ^2-Enoyl CoA hydratases

The long-chain hydratase is part of the membrane-bound **trifunctional enzyme** which is a hetero-octamer of four α- and four β-subunits. The short-chain hydratase (also active with substrates up to C_{16}) is located in the matrix.

3-Hydroxyacyl CoA dehydrogenases

There is considerable overlap of specificity between the membrane-bound **long-chain 3-hydroxyacyl CoA dehydrogenase (LCHAD)**, which is part of the α-subunit of the **trifunctional enzyme**, and the matrix **short-chain hydroxyacyl CoA dehydrogenase (SCHAD)**.

3-Oxoacyl CoA thiolases (ketothiolases)

There are three thiolases: **(i)** a component of the β-subunit of the **trifunctional enzyme**; **(ii)** a **'general' thiolase** found in the matrix with broad activity covering C_6 to C_{16}; and **(iii)** one specific for acetoacetyl CoA.

MCAD and LCHAD deficiency
Sudden infant death syndrome

The sudden unexplained death of an infant while sleeping is known as a 'cot death' or 'sudden infant death syndrome' (SIDS). In a few cases of SIDS a possible cause is deficiency of medium-chain acyl CoA dehydrogenase (MCAD) or long-chain 3-hydroxylacyl CoA dehydrogenase deficiency (LCHAD). In this condition, β-oxidation is restricted and so there is increased oxidation of glucose as a respiratory fuel to meet the demands for energy (see Chapter 6). If the reserves of glycogen become exhausted, this may result in fatal hypoglycaemia.

MCAD deficiency, carnitine deficiency and abnormal metabolites

In MCAD deficiency, there is a tendency for the (C_{10}) acyl CoA, (C_8) acyl CoA, and (C_6) acyl CoA intermediates to accumulate. Accordingly, they are diverted in three directions:

(i) They can be metabolized by ω-oxidation to form the dicarboxylic acids, sebacic acid, suberic acid and adipic acid.

(ii) They can be conjugated with carnitine to form carnitine conjugates, which are excreted in the urine. This urinary loss of carnitine conjugates can cause carnitine deficiency. In turn, this impairs fatty acid transport into the mitochondrion thereby further restricting β-oxidation.

(iii) Suberic acid and hexanoyl CoA can conjugate with glycine to form suberylglycine and hexanoylglycine.

Also, β-oxidation of the unsaturated fatty acid, linoleic acid, produces *cis-*Δ^4-decenoate, which accumulates in MCAD deficiency (see Chapter 29) and is used diagnostically.

Glutaric acidurias

It is convenient to mention these disorders of amino acid metabolism here because of their link with fatty acid metabolism.

Glutaric aciduria I

This condition is due to deficiency of glutaryl CoA dehydrogenase causing an increased excretion of glutarate in the urine.

Glutaric aciduria II (multiple acyl CoA dehydrogenase deficiency, MADD)

In this condition, although glutaryl CoA dehydrogenase is normal, the defect is downstream in the flow of reducing equivalents at the level of ETF or ETF:QO. Because these components are essential for the oxidation of numerous acyl CoA intermediates involved in both amino acid and fatty acid metabolism, this condition has also been called multiple acyl CoA dehydrogenase deficiency (MADD). In particular, glutaryl CoA formed from lysine and tryptophan metabolism accumulates if ETF or ETF:QO are deficient causing glutarate to appear in the urine (see Chart 26.1).

Reference

Eaton S., Bartlett K. & Pourfarzam M. (1996) Review article: Mammalian β-oxidation. *Biochem J,* **320**, 345–57.

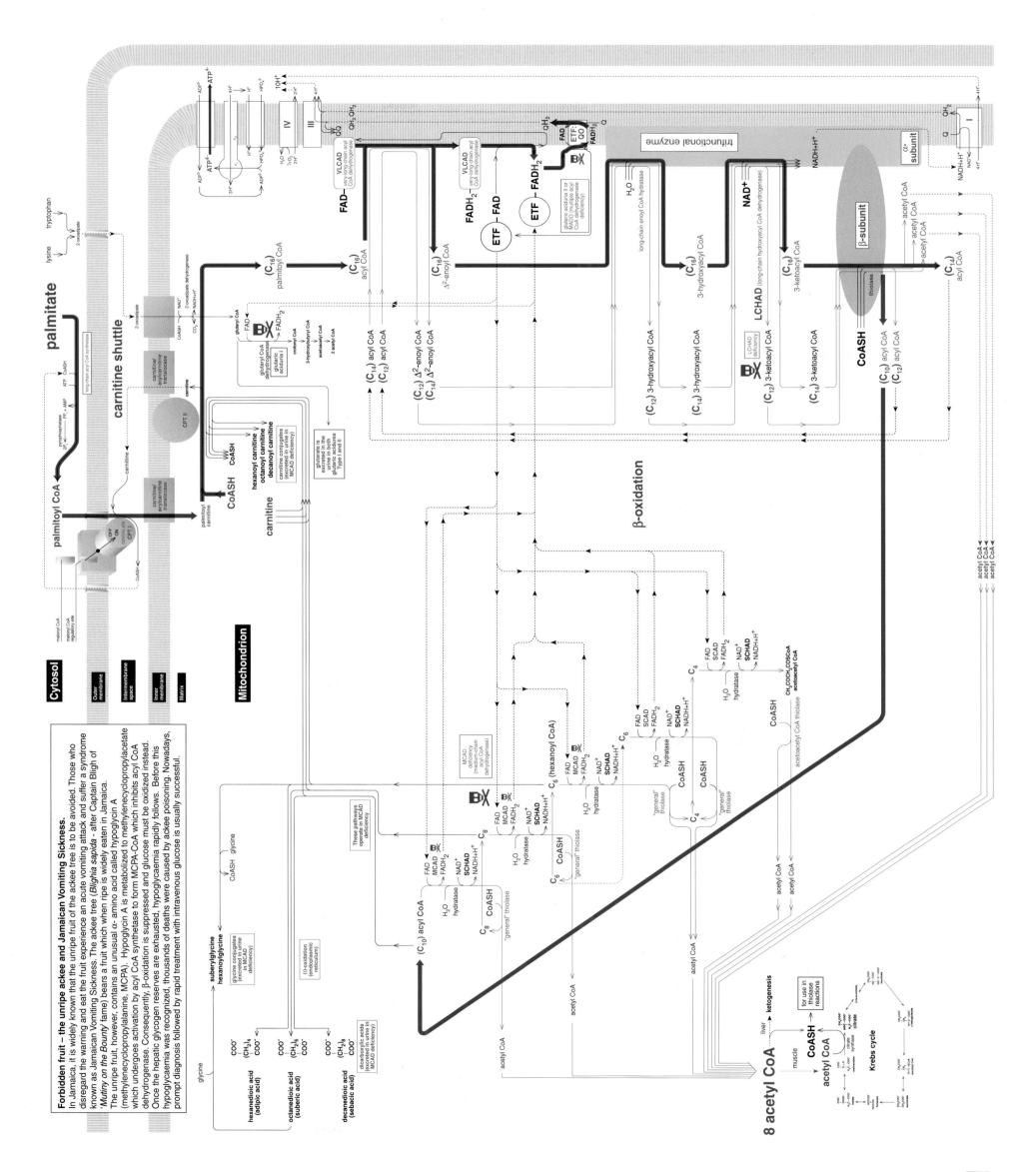

Forbidden fruit – the unripe ackee and Jamaican Vomiting Sickness.
In Jamaica, it is widely known that the unripe fruit of the ackee tree is to be avoided. Those who disregard the warning and eat the fruit experience an acute vomiting attack and suffer a syndrome known as Jamaican Vomiting Sickness. The ackee tree (*Blighia sapida* - after Captain Bligh of '*Mutiny on the Bounty*' fame) bears a fruit which when ripe is widely eaten in Jamaica. The unripe fruit, however, contains an unusual α- amino acid called hypoglycin A (methylenecyclopropylalanine, MCPA). Hypoglycin A is metabolized to methylenecyclopropylacetate which undergoes activation by acyl CoA synthetase to form MCPA-CoA which inhibits acyl CoA dehydrogenase. Consequently, β-oxidation is suppressed and glucose must be oxidized instead. Once the hepatic glycogen reserves are exhausted, hypoglycaemia rapidly follows. Before this hypoglycaemia was recognized, thousands of deaths were caused by ackee poisoning. Nowadays, prompt diagnosis followed by rapid treatment with intravenous glucose is usually successful.

61

The ketone bodies

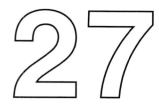

The misunderstood 'villains' of metabolism

Diabetic patients know that the detection in their urine of the 'ketone bodies' (namely D-3-hydroxybutyrate, acetoacetate and acetone) is a danger signal that their diabetes is poorly controlled. Indeed, in severely uncontrolled diabetes, if the ketone bodies are produced in massive supranormal quantities they are associated with ketoacidosis. In this life-threatening complication of diabetes mellitus, the acids D-3-hydroxybutyric acid and acetoacetic acid are produced rapidly, causing high concentrations of protons, which overwhelm the body's acid–base buffering system, with the consequential dangerous decrease in blood pH. It is this low pH due to the protons that is so harmful, and not the ketone bodies themselves.

Until the mid-1960s, it was thought that the ketone bodies were 'metabolic garbage' with no beneficial physiological role. However, it is now realized that, during starvation, the brain uses the ketone bodies as a fuel in addition to its usual fuel glucose. This **regulated and controlled** production of the ketone bodies causes a state known as '**ketosis**'. In ketosis the blood pH remains buffered within normal limits. This is a very important glucose-sparing (and therefore tissue-protein-conserving) adaptation to starvation that compensates for exhaustion of the glycogen reserves. (It should be remembered that the brain cannot use fatty acids as a fuel.)

Chart 27.1: Ketogenesis

During starvation, prolonged severe exercise or uncontrolled diabetes, the rate of production of the ketone bodies is increased. The most important precursors for ketogenesis are fatty acids derived from triacylglycerols. However, certain amino acids (leucine, isoleucine, lysine, phenylalanine, tyrosine and tryptophan) are also ketogenic.

Ketogenesis from triacylglycerols

The ketone bodies are produced in liver mitochondria from **fatty acids**, which in turn are produced by the action of **hormone-sensitive lipase** on **triacylglycerols** stored in adipose tissue. The fatty acids are subjected to β-oxidation to form **acetyl CoA**. The interdependent relationship between the pathways for β-oxidation and gluconeogenesis is emphasized in Chapter 23 and is illustrated in Chart 27.1, which shows how mitochondrial

oxaloacetate is diverted towards gluconeogenesis. Hence, oxaloacetate, which is needed by the **citrate synthase** reaction for acetyl CoA to enter Krebs cycle, is directed away from the mitochondrion to the cytosol for gluconeogenesis. Consequently, there is an increased flux of acetyl CoA through **acetoacetyl CoA thiolase** towards ketogenesis.

Ketogenesis involves the **acetoacetyl CoA thiolase** reaction, which combines two molecules of acetyl CoA to form **acetoacetyl CoA**. This in turn is condensed with a third acetyl CoA by **HMGCoA synthase** to form 3-hydroxy-3-methylglutaryl-CoA (**HMGCoA**) (see Chart 27.1). Finally, HMGCoA is cleaved by **HMGCoA-lyase** to form **acetoacetate** and acetyl CoA. The NADH formed by the L-3-hydroxyacyl CoA dehydrogenase reaction of β-oxidation could be coupled to the reduction of acetoacetate to D-3-hydroxybutyrate, thereby regenerating NAD+. Acetone is produced by non-enzymic decarboxylation of acetoacetate, and is formed in relatively small proportions compared with the acids.

The rate of ketogenesis is coupled to the supply of fatty acids and the regulation of β-oxidation, as described in Chapters 25 & 26.

The ketone bodies are thought to leave the mitochondrion by a carrier mechanism in exchange for pyruvate.

Ketogenesis from amino acids

Certain amino acids can wholly or partially be used for ketogenesis. The details of these pathways are shown in Chapters 36 & 37. Entry to ketogenesis is at acetyl CoA (isoleucine), acetoacetate (phenylalanine and tyrosine), HMGCoA (leucine) or acetoacetyl CoA (lysine and tryptophan), as outlined in Chart 27.1.

Diagram 27.1: Fatty acids are mobilized from adipose tissue for ketogenesis in the liver

In the ketotic state, hormone-sensitive lipase is active and triacylglycerols are hydrolysed to glycerol and fatty acids. The liberated fatty acids leave the adipocyte and diffuse into the blood, where they are bound to albumin and transported to the liver. In the liver, β-oxidation and ketogenesis occur. The 'ketone bodies' acetoacetate and D-3-hydroxybutyrate produced are exported as fuel for tissue oxidation, especially by muscle and by the brain.

Diagram 27.1 Fatty acid mobilization from adipose tissue for ketogenesis in the liver.

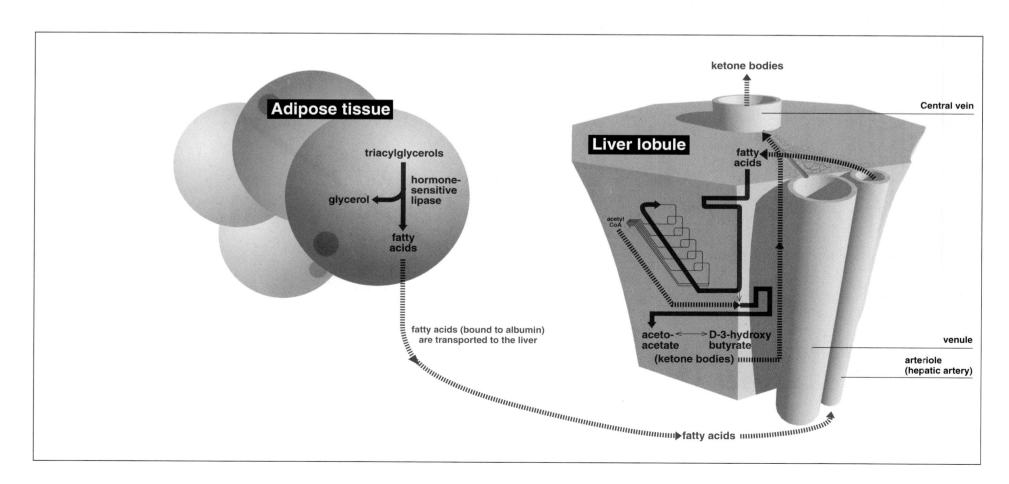

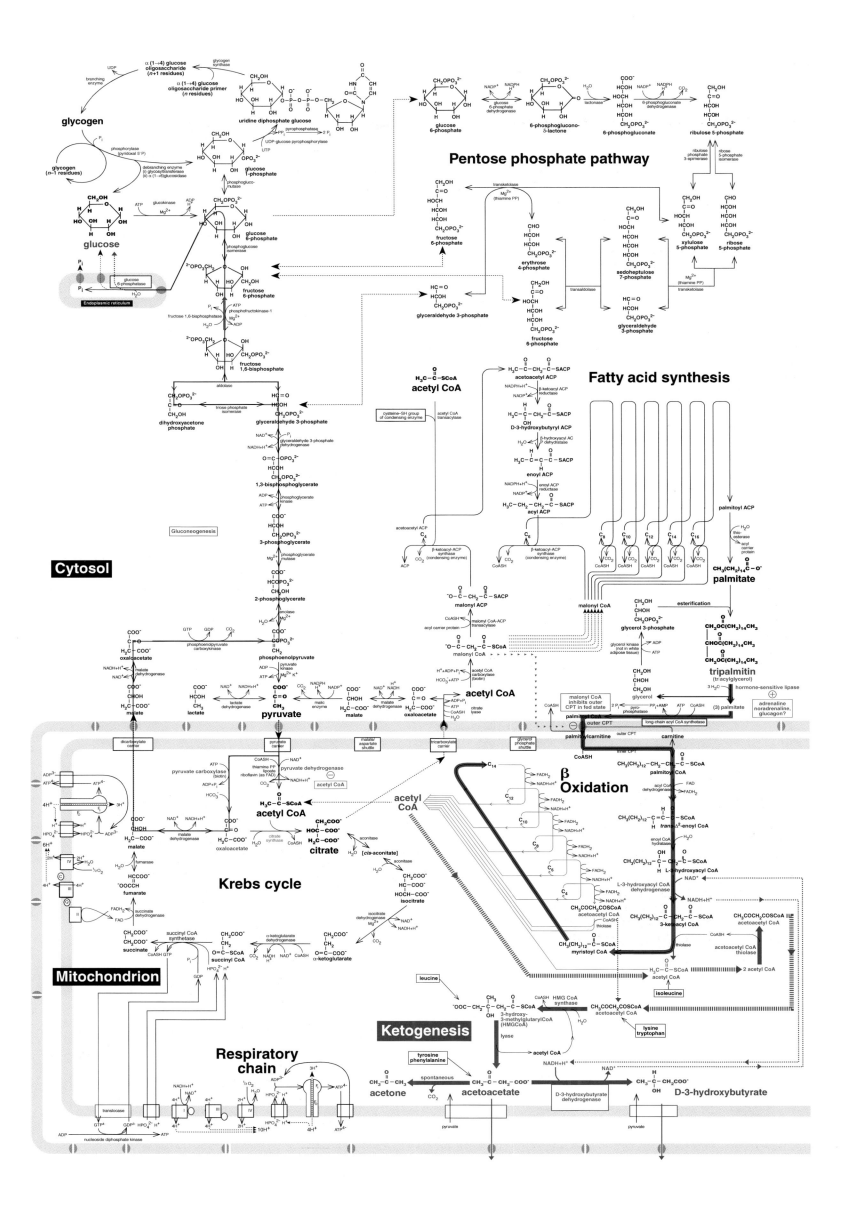

Chart 27.1 Ketogenesis.

Ketone body utilization

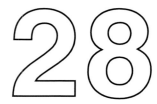

The ketone bodies are an important fuel for the brain during starvation

The brain has an enormous need for respiratory fuel, each day requiring approximately 140 g of glucose, which is equivalent to nearly 600 kcal (it should be remembered that brain cannot use fatty acids as a fuel). The large quantities of ATP produced are needed by the sodium pump mechanism, which maintains the membrane potentials, which in turn are essential for the conduction of nerve impulses. Clearly, to stay alive, the brain must be supplied with respiratory fuel at all times!

During starvation, once the glycogen reserves are exhausted, the rate at which ketone bodies are produced from fatty acids by the liver is increased so they can be used by tissues, but particularly the brain, to generate ATP. Consequently, the use of glucose as a fuel by the brain is considerably reduced. The advantage of switching to the ketone bodies for energy is because, during starvation, glucose is obtained by gluconeogenesis from muscle protein. This causes wasting of the muscles and so the 'glucose-sparing' effect of the ketone bodies is an important adaptation to the stress of starvation.

Chart 28.1: Utilization of ketone bodies

The ketone bodies are first converted to acetyl CoA, which can then be oxidized by the Krebs cycle. The enzymes needed are **δ-3-hydroxybutyrate dehydrogenase, 3-ketoacyl CoA transferase** and **acetoacetyl CoA thiolase**. It should be noted that the 3-ketoacyl CoA transferase is not found in liver. Consequently, the liver is unable to use the ketone bodies as respiratory fuel. On the other hand, although several tissues are capable of ketone utilization – notably muscle and kidney – ketone bodies are particularly important as a fuel for brain and other nerve cells during starvation.

As illustrated in Chart 28.1 opposite, D-3-hydroxybutyrate dehydrogenase is bound to the inner mitochondrial membrane, where it catalyses the formation of acetoacetate from D-3-hydroxybutyrate. Then, in the presence of 3-ketoacyl-CoA transferase, CoA is transferred from succinyl CoA to form acetoacetyl CoA. Subsequently, in the presence of CoA and acetoacetyl CoA

thiolase, acetoacetyl CoA is cleaved to yield two molecules of acetyl CoA for oxidation in Krebs cycle.

ATP yield from the complete oxidation of D-3-hydroxybutyrate

NB: The calculation below uses the 'non-integral' values for P/O ratios (see Chapter 3). The oxidation of D-3-hydroxybutyrate generates two molecules of acetyl CoA, which yield a net total equivalent to 21.25 molecules of ATP as follows:

	ATP yield
D-3-hydroxybutyrate dehydrogenase	
1 NADH	2.5
Krebs cycle	
6 NADH	15
2 FADH$_2$	3
Succinyl CoA synthetase (via GTP)	1
But, one H$^+$ is used by the phosphate carrier	
This is equivalent to loss of 0·25 ATP	−0.25
Total	**21.25 ATP**

Similarly, acetoacetate can generate a total equivalent to 18.75 molecules of ATP.

It should be noted that one of the pair of succinyl CoA molecules is temporarily diverted from Krebs cycle for the 3-ketoacyl CoA transferase reaction, where it 'activates' acetoacetate. This energy is therefore not available for ATP synthesis. The succinate liberated is, however, free to return to Krebs cycle for further oxidation.

In comparison with glucose, the ketone bodies are a very good respiratory fuel. Whereas 100 g of glucose generates 8.7 kg of ATP, 100 g of D-3-hydroxybutyrate can yield 10.5 kg ATP, and 100 g of acetoacetate produces 9.4 kg of ATP.

Diagram 28.1 A generalized scheme representing the delivery of glucose and ketone bodies to nerve cells.

The diagram shows the relationship of a capillary to a non-myelinated and a myelinated axon. Electron microscopy has demonstrated that, in myelinated axons, small clusters of mitochondria occur at the node of Ranvier. It is most probable that in myelinated axons the glucose transporters will also be located at these nodes, which are very metabolically active. On the other hand, in non-myelinated axons, mitochondria and glucose transporters are probably distributed uniformly along the length of the axon.

In both types of axon, glucose and the ketone bodies diffuse from the capillary, through the axolemma (via the GLUT3 glucose transporter) and into the axoplasm for metabolism.

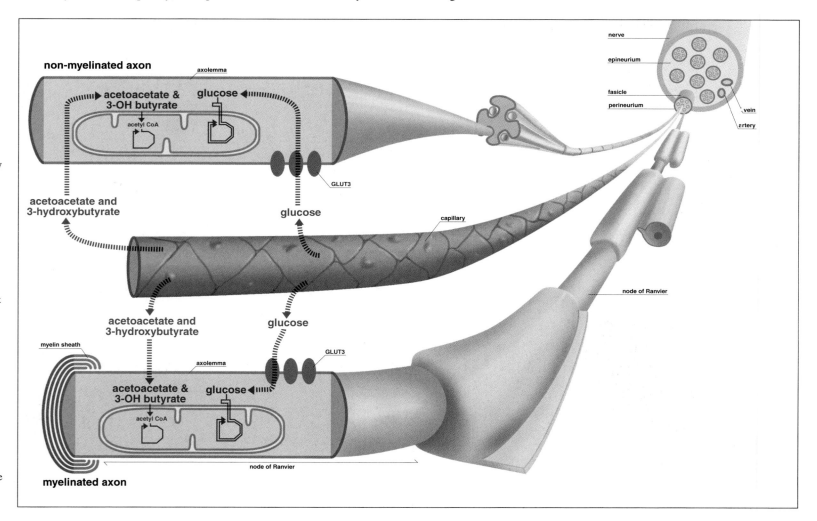

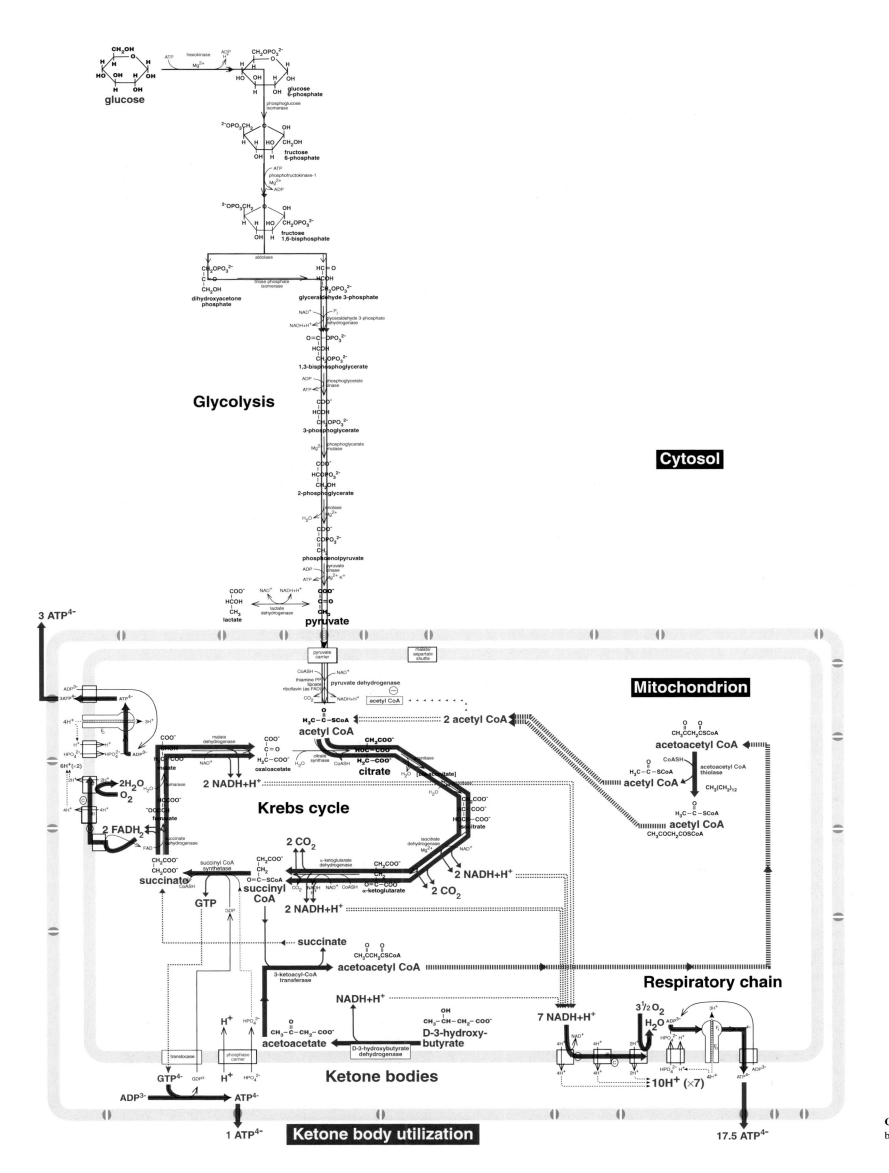

Chart 28.1 Ketone body utilization.

β-Oxidation of unsaturated fatty acids

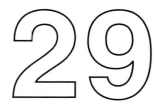

The naturally occurring unsaturated fatty acids have double bonds in the *cis*-configuration, but β-oxidation, as described in Chapter 15, produces intermediates with the *trans*-configuration. This stereoisomeric complication means that β-oxidation of unsaturated fatty acids requires two additional enzymes: **3,2-enoyl CoA isomerase**, and **2,4-dienoyl CoA reductase**.

Chart 29.1: β-Oxidation of linoleic acid

The β-oxidation of the polyunsaturated fatty acid, linoleic acid, is illustrated in Chart 29.1, which demonstrates the similarities and differences in comparison with the saturated fatty acid derivative, palmitoyl CoA (see Chart 15.1 and Chapter 26). The oxidation of unsaturated fatty acids is relatively slow compared with saturated fatty acids because the former are transported slowly into mitochondria by the **carnitine shuttle** (Chaper 26).

Cycles 1–3

The first three cycles of β-oxidation, whereby linoleate ($C_{18:2}$) is shortened to dodecadienoate ($C_{12:2}$) via $C_{16:2}$ and $C_{14:2}$, are identical to the reactions for saturated fatty acids described in Chapters 15 and 26.

Cycle 4 requires 3,2-enoyl CoA isomerase (*cis*-Δ^3 [or *trans*-Δ^3] → *trans*-Δ^2-enoyl CoA isomerase)

The all *cis*-$C_{12:2}$ product (*cis*-Δ^3, *cis*-Δ^6-dodecadienoyl CoA), is not a substrate for enoyl CoA hydratase. The enzyme 3,2-enoyl CoA isomerase catalyses conversion of the *cis*-Δ^3 double bond to a *trans*-Δ^2 double bond. The hydration of the resulting *trans*-Δ^2-enoyl CoA is mediated by enoyl CoA hydratase. The dehydrogenase and thiolase reactions subsequently produce ($C_{10:1}$) *cis*-Δ^4-decenoyl CoA and acetyl CoA.

Cycle 5 requires both a 'novel' reductase and the isomerase

Cycle 5 begins with ($C_{10:1}$) *cis*-Δ^4-decenoyl CoA, which is oxidized as usual by acyl CoA dehydrogenase. However, the *cis*-Δ^4 double bond of the

trans-Δ^2- *cis*-Δ^4 product inhibits the hydratase reaction. A recently discovered enzyme, **2,4-dienoyl CoA reductase**, catalyses the reduction of this metabolite by NADPH to form the *trans*-Δ^3-enoyl CoA intermediate. This is then isomerized by the versatile 3,2-isomerase, which changes the *trans*-Δ^3- to the *trans*-Δ^2-enoyl CoA form, which is a substrate for enoyl CoA hydratase. The usual sequence of β-oxidation reactions catalysed by the dehydrogenase and thiolase then produce ($C_{8:0}$) octanoyl CoA.

Cycles 6–8

Since ($C_{8:0}$) octanoyl CoA is fully saturated, it is oxidized by the familiar β-oxidation pathway to yield acetyl CoA.

What about the epimerase reaction?

Several textbooks describe the need for a '3-hydroxyacyl CoA epimerase' in the pathway for the β-oxidation of unsaturated fatty acids. This is because it used to be thought that enoyl CoA hydratase added water across a *cis*-Δ^2 double bond to form the D-isomer of hydroxyacyl CoA, i.e. not the L-isomer needed for L-3-hydroxyacyl CoA dehydrogenase. The epimerase was thought to be needed to invert the configuration of the hydroxyl group at C_3 from the D-isomer to the L-isomer, thereby providing a suitable substrate for the L-3-hydroxyacyl CoA dehydrogenase.

Current opinion is that the epimerase is not in the mitochondria but is instead found in the peroxisomes. Indeed, there is evidence to suggest that this 'epimerase' activity is due to the reactions of two distinct 2-enoyl CoA hydratases recently discovered in peroxisomes.

Fatty acid nomenclature

This is complicated and a knowledge of Greek helps. The various elements involved in the naming of fatty acids are summarized in Diagram 29.1.

Diagram 29.1 Fatty acid nomenclature. **NB**: Although the compounds shown could exist in theory, relatively few are known to occur in nature except as metabolic intermediates.

Number of carbon atoms present	Prefix C_6	C_8	C_{10}	C_{12}	C_{14}	C_{16}	C_{18}	C_{20}	C_{22}	C_{24}	C_{26}	Suffix
Number of carbon-to-carbon double-bonds present nil	hexan...	octan...	decan...	dodecan...	tetradecan...	hexadecan...	octadecan...	eicosan...	docosan...	tetracosan...	hexacosan...	...oic
1	hexen...	octen...	decen...	dodecen...	tetradecen...	hexadecen...	octadecen...	eicosen...	docosen...	tetracosen...	hexacosen...	...oic
2	hexa...	octa...	deca...	dodeca...	tetradeca...	hexadeca...	octadeca...	eicosa...	docosa...	tetracosa...	hexacosa...	...dienoic
3		octa...	deca...	dodeca...	tetradeca...	hexadeca...	octadeca...	eicosa...	docosa...	tetracosa...	hexacosa...	...trienoic
4			deca...	dodeca...	tetradeca...	hexadeca...	octadeca...	eicosa...	docosa...	tetracosa...	hexacosa...	...tetraenoic
5				dodeca...	tetradeca...	hexadeca...	octadeca...	eicosa...	docosa...	tetracosa...	hexacosa...	...pentaenoic
6					tetradeca...	hexadeca...	octadeca...	eicosa...	docosa...	tetracosa...	hexacosa...	...hexaenoic

Identification of carbon atoms

Numbering from carboxyl carbon atom	10	9	8	7	6	5	4	3	2	1
Greek letters	ω				ε	δ	γ	β	α	
Numbering from ω carbon atom	ω1	ω2	ω3	ω4	ω5	ω6				
Numbering from n carbon atom (methyl group)	n-1	n-2	n-3	n-4	n-5	n-6				

CH₃ .... COOH

Identification of double bonds

Double bonds. Symbolized by Δ and superscript representing position
  ω-family. Indicates position of double bond from the methyl end
  n-family. Indentical to above — a more modern convention
Isomeric form. *cis*- or *trans*- (the convention preferred by biochemists)
or, *Z* or *E* (the convention preferred by chemists)

Δ^4- Δ^2-
ω6
n-6
cis-   *trans*-
Z   *E*

Summary

The fatty acid shown above is named as follows:
Length of carbon chain is **10** carbon atoms, C_{10}
There are two **2** carbon-to-carbon double-bonds present. $C_{10:2}$
Hence the above example is a $C_{10:2}$ unsaturated fatty acid, namely *trans*-Δ^2-, *cis*-Δ^4-**decadienoic acid**
which is a **n-6** (or alternatively ω6) unsaturated fatty acid.
NB: This is not a common, naturally occurring fatty acid. However, its thioester with CoA is formed during the β-oxidation of linoleic acid (see Chart opposite)

Confusion! The α- and γ- prefixes of α- and γ-linolenate are **not** based on the above conventions.

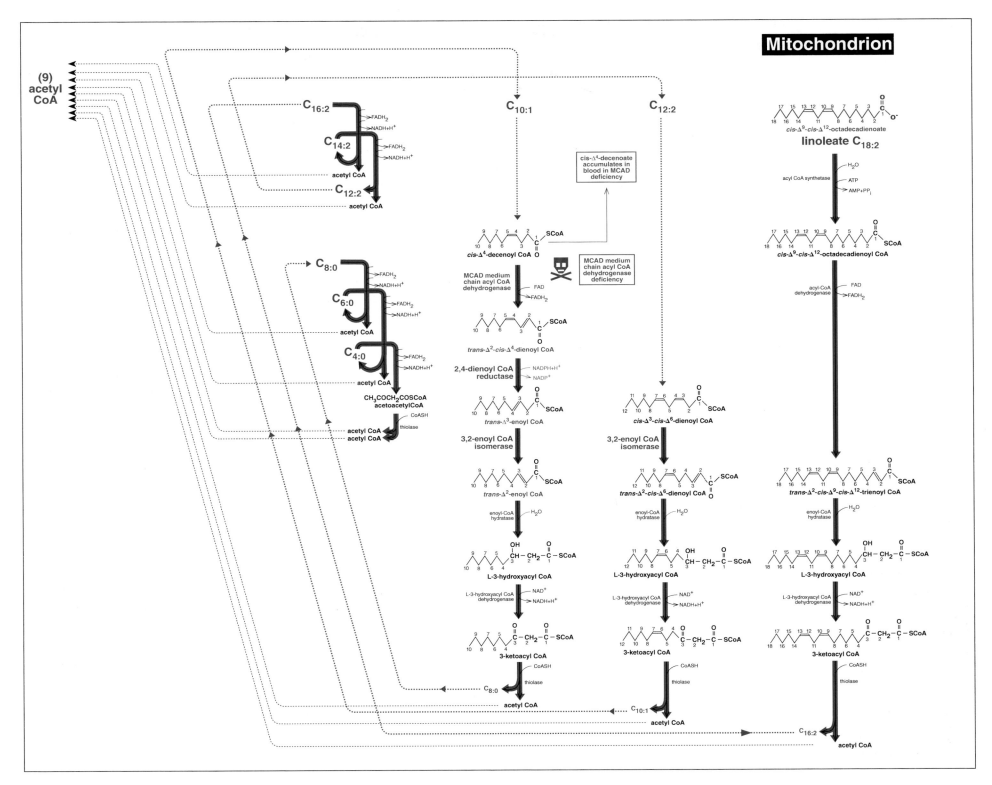

Chart 29.1 β-Oxidation of linoleic acid ($C_{18:2}$ n-6). In medium-chain acyl CoA dehydrogenase deficiency (MCAD), ***cis-*Δ^4*-decenoate** accumulates in the blood, and the finding of increased levels in a patient is used in the diagnosis of this condition, see Chapter 26.

Peroxisomal β-oxidation

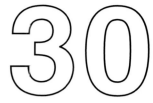

Mitochondria are not the only location for β-oxidation

The pathway for the β-oxidation of fatty acids was once thought to be restricted exclusively to mitochondria. However, mammalian peroxisomal β-oxidation of fatty acids was confirmed in 1976 by Lazarow and de Duve. Peroxisomal β-oxidation occurs in both the liver and kidney. It is now thought that approximately 90% of short- and medium-chain fatty acids are oxidized in the mitochondria, whilst approximately 10% are oxidized in the peroxisomes in the basal state. However, under conditions of induced proliferation of the peroxisomes, whether by drugs (e.g. clofibrate) or a high-fat diet, the relative importance of peroxisomal β-oxidation is substantially increased.

Whereas the structural changes in the metabolic intermediates formed during β-oxidation are chemically identical in both the peroxisomes and mitochondria, different and distinct enzymes are involved in the two organelles. An important difference in peroxisomal β-oxidation is that it is much more versatile than the mitochondrial pathway. It is capable of metabolizing a wide variety of fatty acid analogues, notably dicarboxylic acids and prostaglandins. However, current opinion is that the main function of peroxisomal β-oxidation is for chain-shortening of very-long-chain fatty acids (i.e. C_{22} and longer) in preparation for their subsequent oxidation by mitochondria. It should be noted that very-long-chain fatty acids cannot enter mitochondria by the carnitine shuttle.

Chart 30.1: Chain-shortening of very-long-chain fatty acids by peroxisomal β-oxidation

The distinguishing features of peroxisomal β-oxidation can be seen in the chart, using C_{24} lignocerate as an example:

1 **Activation.** A **very-long-chain acyl CoA synthetase**, which is located on the cytosolic side of the peroxisomal membrane, activates the fatty acid to form **lignoceroyl CoA**.

2 **Transport across peroxisomal membrane.** The peroxisomal membrane contains a **peroxisomal membrane protein**, which enables the lignoceroyl CoA to diffuse across it by passive transport. It also allows the products of β-oxidation to diffuse out of the peroxisome.

3 **Oxidation of fatty acids.** In peroxisomes, the first oxidation step is catalysed by the FAD-containing enzyme **acyl CoA oxidase. NB:** This reaction, in which the electrons are passed directly to oxygen, is insensitive to the respiratory chain inhibitor, cyanide (see Chapter 3). The hydrogen peroxide formed is broken down to water and oxygen in the presence of **catalase**. Note also that, in contrast to mitochondrial β-oxidation which employs FAD-dependent acyl CoA dehydrogenase, ATP is not formed in peroxisomes at this stage and instead the energy is dissipated as heat.

4 **Bifunctional enzyme.** The bifunctional enzyme has both **enoyl CoA hydratase** and **L-3-hydroxyacyl CoA dehydrogenase** activity. The dehydrogenase forms NADH, the accumulation of which could become rate-limiting. The fate of NADH depends on the energy status of the cell. It could in theory pass into the mitochondrion via the malate–aspartate shuttle. Alternatively, evidence using isolated rat liver peroxisomes suggests that the **lactate dehydrogenase** reaction could be important for the reoxidation of NADH, as shown in the chart.

5 **The products of peroxisomal β-oxidation.** The products of chain shortening are **acetyl CoA** and the newly formed acyl CoA (i.e. palmitoyl CoA, as shown in Chart 30.1). The precise details of their subsequent fate are not yet clear. In principle, both of these could leave the peroxisome unchanged, or they could be hydrolysed by peroxisomal hydrolase to acetate, or to their free acyl derivatives. Another possibility is that acylcarnitine might be formed in the peroxisome prior to export to the mitochondria for further β-oxidation. Because of this uncertainty, the representation in the chart should be regarded as a simplification.

Peroxisomal β-oxidation of unsaturated fatty acids and the 'trifunctional' enzyme

The mitochondrial β-oxidation of unsaturated fatty acids is described in Chapter 29. However, there is now evidence which suggests that some unsaturated fatty acids are readily metabolized by peroxisomal β-oxidation. Accordingly, peroxisomes have a **2,4-dienoyl CoA reductase**. They also have **3,2-enoyl CoA isomerase activity** (see Chapter 29). Indeed, there is evidence to suggest that the latter is associated with the 'bifunctional' enzyme, thereby conferring upon it 'trifunctional' status.

Saturated

Notional name	Systematic name	Common name	
$C_{6:0}$	hexanoic acid	caproic acid	Latin *caper* goat
$C_{8:0}$	octanoic acid	caprylic acid	Latin *caper* goat
$C_{10:0}$	decanoic acid	capric acid	Found in butter, coconut oil etc
$C_{12:0}$	dodecanoic acid	lauric acid	Found in berries of laurel
$C_{14:0}$	tetradecanoic acid	myristic acid	*Myristica* : nutmeg tree (found in nutmeg oil etc.)
$C_{16:0}$	hexadecanoic acid	palmitic acid	Found in palm oil
$C_{18:0}$	octadecanoic acid	stearic acid	Greek *stear* fat
$C_{20:0}$	eicosanoic acid	arachidic acid	*Arachis* : peanut
$C_{22:0}$	docosanoic acid	behenic acid	In oil of ben, seed oil of the horse-radish tree, *Moringa pterygospermum*
$C_{24:0}$	tetracosanoic acid	lignoceric acid	Latin *lignum* wood (found in beech-wood tar)
$C_{26:0}$	hexacosanoic acid	cerotic acid	Greek *keros* wax
$C_{28:0}$	octacosanoic acid	montanic acid	In montan wax (extracted from lignite)

Unsaturated

Notional name	Systematic name	Common name	
$C_{4:1}$	*trans*-Δ^2-tetraenoic acid	crotonic acid	Greek *kroton* castor-oil plant.
$C_{16:1}$n-7	*cis*-Δ^9-hexadecenoic acid	palmitoleic acid	Palm oil
$C_{18:1}$n-9	*cis*-Δ^9-octadecenoic acid	oleic acid	Latin *oleum* oil
$C_{18:1}$n-7	*cis*-Δ^{11}-octadecenoic acid	vaccenic acid	Latin *vacca* cow (in beef fat)
$C_{18:2}$n-6	all *cis*-$\Delta^{9,12}$-octadecadienoate	linoleic acid	Latin *linum* flax, and *oleum* oil (in linseed oil etc)
$C_{18:3}$n-3	all *cis*-$\Delta^{9,12,15}$-octadecatrienoic acid	α-linolenic acid	
$C_{18:3}$n-6	all *cis*-$\Delta^{6,9,12}$-octadecatrienoic acid	GLA (γ-linolenic acid)	GLA (Found in evening primrose oil)
$C_{20:1}$n-9	*cis*-Δ^{11}-eicosenoic acid	gondoic acid	
$C_{20:4}$n-6	all *cis*-$\Delta^{5,8,11,14}$-eicosatetraenoic acid	arachidonic acid	*Arachis* : peanut
$C_{20:5}$n-3	all *cis*-$\Delta^{5,8,11,14,17}$-eicosapentaenoic acid	EPA (timnodonic acid)	Eicosapentaenoic acid (found in fish oil)
$C_{22:1}$n-9	*cis*-Δ^{13}-docosenoic acid	erucic acid	Latin *eruca* cabbage (in seed oil of *Cruciferae* : mustard, rape etc.)
$C_{22:5}$n-3	all *cis*-$\Delta^{7,10,13,16,19}$-docosapentaenoic acid	clupanodonic acid	*Clupeidae* herring (found in fish oil)
$C_{22:6}$n-3	all *cis*-$\Delta^{4,7,10,13,16,19}$-docosahexaenoic acid	DHA (cervonic acid)	Docosahexaenoic acid (found in fish oil)

Diagram 30.1 Nomenclature of some naturally occurring fatty acids.

Adrenoleukodystrophy and Lorenzo's Oil

X-linked adrenoleukodystrophy (ALD) is a disorder of peroxisomal β-oxidation which results in the accumulation of very-long-chain fatty acids especially $C_{24:0}$ (lignoceric acid) and $C_{26:0}$ (cerotic acid). It was once thought the disease was due to a deficiency of very-long-chain acyl CoA synthetase, but recent evidence suggests the gene encodes a peroxisomal membrane protein (ALDP) which is thought to be involved in the uptake of very-long-chain acyl CoA precursors into the peroxisome for β-oxidation.

Adrenoleukodystrophy was drawn to public attention by Lorenzo Odone who was diagnosed with the condition as featured in the film *Lorenzo's Oil* released in 1993 by Universal Studios. The remarkable perseverence of his parents, Augusto and Michaela Odone, who were not biochemists, led to the discovery that glyceryl trierucate ($C_{22:1}$) and glyceryl trioleate ($C_{18:1}$) dramatically lowered blood levels of very-long-chain fatty acids. This formulation, known as 'Lorenzo's Oil', is being studied in worldwide trials to establish its efficacy in the treatment of ALD.

This formulation, known as "Lorenzo's Oil", has been the subject of worldwide trials. Unfortunately, Lorenzo's oil does not protect the development of childhood ALD. However, preliminary data suggest that the progression of the disease may be altered if treatment is started in asymptomatic boys less than five years old but longer term follow-up is needed to confirm these findings.

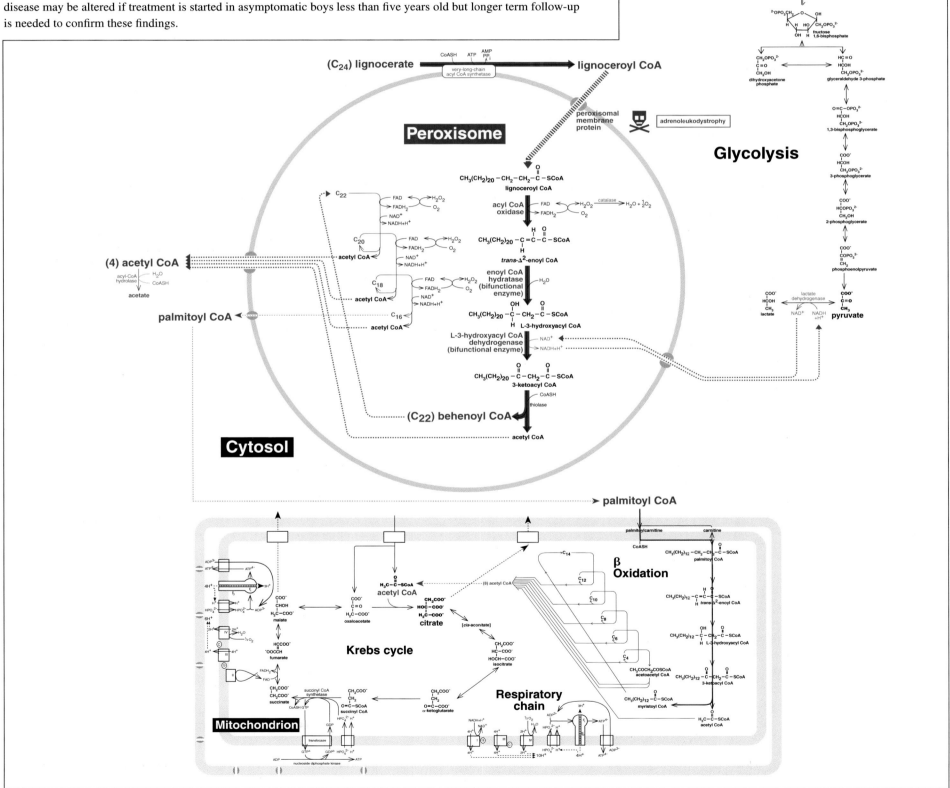

Chart 30.1 Peroxisomal β-oxidation of lignoceric acid.

Elongation and desaturation of fatty acids

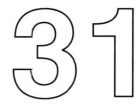

We have seen in Chapter 11 how ($C_{16:0}$) palmitate and ($C_{18:0}$) stearate, are formed by the fatty acid synthase complex. These products can be modified in various ways. Additional carbon atoms can be added to form long-chain fatty acids. Alternatively, or as well, fatty acids can be desaturated to yield products with one or more double bonds. The long-chain polyunsaturated fatty acids so formed are used for synthesizing membrane phospholipids and the prostaglandins.

Elongation of fatty acids by the endoplasmic reticulum pathway

An example of chain elongation followed by desaturation is shown in Chart 31.1 opposite. Here ($C_{18:3}$) γ-linolenic acid is initially lengthened to ($C_{20:3}$) dihomo-γ-linolenoyl CoA, which is desaturated to ($C_{20:4}$) arachidonoyl CoA.

The endoplasmic reticulum pathway by which fatty acids are elongated is similar to the pathway for fatty acid synthesis described in Chapter 11. The principal differences are:

1 For chain elongation, the two NADPH-dependent **reductase** enzymes and the **dehydratase** are located on the cytosolic surface of the smooth endoplasmic reticulum.

2 Instead of acyl carrier protein (ACP), the intermediates for chain elongation are bound to CoA.

3 The 2-carbon donor is **malonyl CoA** (not malonyl-ACP).

Desaturation of fatty acids

Mammals have three desaturases: Δ^5-, Δ^6- and Δ^9-fatty acyl CoA desaturases. These enzymes have a broad chain-length specificity and occur mainly in liver. **NB:** Previous reports of Δ^4-desaturase activity are now in doubt (see opposite).

A wide range of different fatty acids can be produced by a combination of the elongation and desaturase reactions. For example, in the chart opposite, Δ^5-**desaturase** is used to form **arachidonic acid**, whereas in Diagram 31.1, the Δ^9-**desaturase** is shown oxidizing ($C_{16:0}$) palmitoyl CoA to ($C_{16:1}$) palmitoleoyl CoA.

The desaturase system, which is located in the membrane of the smooth endoplasmic reticulum, consists of the **desaturase(s)**, **cytochrome b_5** and **cytochrome b_5 reductase**.

Diagram 31.1: The desaturation of palmitoyl CoA to form palmitoleoyl CoA

Diagram 31.1 The desaturation of palmitoyl CoA to form palmitoleoyl CoA.

The diagram illustrates the desaturation of palmitoyl CoA to palmitoleoyl CoA. It should be noted that molecular oxygen is the terminal electron acceptor and that it receives **two** pairs of electrons: one originating from the 9,10 double bond of palmitoyl CoA and the second donated by NADH.

Let us first consider the electrons derived from the 9,10 C–H bond of palmitoyl CoA in the reaction catalysed by Δ^9-**desaturase**. The desaturases are enzymes that contain non-haem ferric iron (Fe^{3+}). The electrons reduce two atoms of this to the ferrous (Fe^{2+}) state prior to the electrons being passed on to oxygen, which combines with $2H^+$ to form water.

Next, consider the electrons provided by NADH. A pair of electrons is donated to the FAD prosthetic group of **cytochrome b_5 reductase**, which is consequently reduced to $FADH_2$. The electrons are then accepted by **cytochrome b_5**, which in turn donates the electrons to oxygen, which combines with $2H^+$ to form water.

Elongation of short-chain fatty acids occurs in mitochondria

The mitochondrial pathway for chain elongation is essentially a reversal of β-oxidation with one exception. The last step in elongation, i.e. the reaction catalysed by **enoyl CoA reductase**, requires NADPH for elongation (see Chart 31.1), whereas the corresponding enzyme for β-oxidation, acyl CoA dehydrogenase, requires FAD (see Chapter 15). The mitochondrial pathway appears to be important for elongating fatty acids containing 14 or fewer carbon atoms. In the chart opposite, this is exemplified by the elongation of ($C_{14:0}$) myristoyl CoA to form ($C_{16:0}$) palmitoyl CoA.

Essential fatty acids

As mentioned earlier, higher mammals, including humans, have enzymes capable of desaturating fatty acids at the Δ^5-, Δ^6- and Δ^9- positions. However, they are incapable of desaturation beyond the C_9 carbon atom. Nevertheless, certain polyunsaturated fatty acids are vital for maintaining health, in particular the 'n-6 family' members, dihomo-γ-linolenic acid and arachidonic acid. These are 20-carbon-chain fatty acids that are precursors of the eicosanoid hormones (Greek *eikosi*, twenty), i.e. the prostaglandins, thromboxanes and leukotrienes, which contain 20 carbon atoms. Accordingly, the 'n-6 family' precursor linoleic acid ($C_{18:2}$, all *cis*-$\Delta^{9,12}$), for example, is essential in the diet and is known as an 'essential fatty acid'. After sequential Δ^6-desaturation, 2-carbon chain elongation, and Δ^5-desaturation, linoleic acid is transformed to arachidonic acid.

Evening primrose and starflower oils: 'the elixir of life'?

Normally, given a healthy diet, linoleic acid is an adequate precursor of its family of polyunsaturated fatty acids. There are circumstances, however, possibly including diabetes mellitus, where Δ^6-desaturase activity is relatively inactive, which limits the conversion of linoleic acid to dihomo-γ-linolenic acid and arachidonic acid. Although controversial, clinical trials suggest that dietary supplementation with γ-linolenic acid ($C_{18:3}$, all *cis*-$\Delta^{6,9,12}$) is beneficial in preventing and minimizing many of the complications of diabetes. Indeed, evening primrose and starflower oils, which are rich in γ-linolenic acid, are currently enjoying a reputation for a wide range of health benefits. As illustrated in Chart 31.1 opposite, γ-linolenic acid is independent of Δ^6-desaturase to form the polyunsaturated products, since it requires only elongation and Δ^5-desaturation.

Therapeutic benefits of evening primrose oil, starflower oil and fish oils

The γ-linolenic acid in evening primrose oil and starflower oil, is, via dihomo-γ-linolenic acid, a precursor of the series 1 prostaglandins. Fish oils are rich in the n-3 fatty acid eicosapentanoic acid, EPA, which is a precursor of the prostaglandin 3 series. It is known that, out of the different prostaglandins, the series 2 prostaglandins have the most potent inflammatory effects, sometimes with pathological consequences. Dietary supplementation with γ-linolenic acid or eicosapentanoic acid causes proportionally enhanced production of the benign series 1 and 3 prostaglandins, thereby displacing the potent inflammatory effects of the 2 series. Clinical trials with these oils have shown beneficial effects in the treatment of inflammatory diseases such as psoriasis and rheumatoid arthritis.

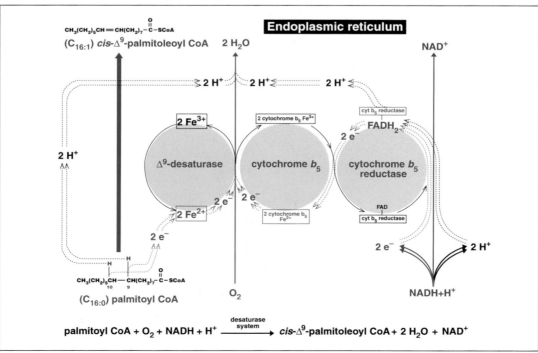

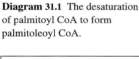

Is there a Δ⁴-desaturase?

Recent evidence suggests that, contrary to previous dogma, microsomes do not possess Δ^4-desaturase activity. However, Δ^4-desaturation can occur by mystical molecular manoeuvering meritworthy of a magician. This involves the cooperation of the endoplasmic reticulum and, probably, the peroxisomes. First of all the long-chain fatty acid designated for Δ^4-desaturation is **chain-lengthened by two** carbon groups. Cunningly, Δ^6-desaturation then occurs and the Δ^6 very-long-chain fatty acid is exported for partial chain-shortening (2 carbon groups) by peroxisomal β-oxidation. Thus, abracadabra, the resulting fatty acid, having been reduced by two carbons, is now a Δ^4-desaturated fatty acid which is returned to the endoplasmic reticulum for phospholipid synthesis.

See, for example, Mohammed B.S. *et al.* (1997) Regulation of the biosynthesis of 4,7,10,13,16-docosapentaenoic acid. *J Biochem,* **326**, 425–30.

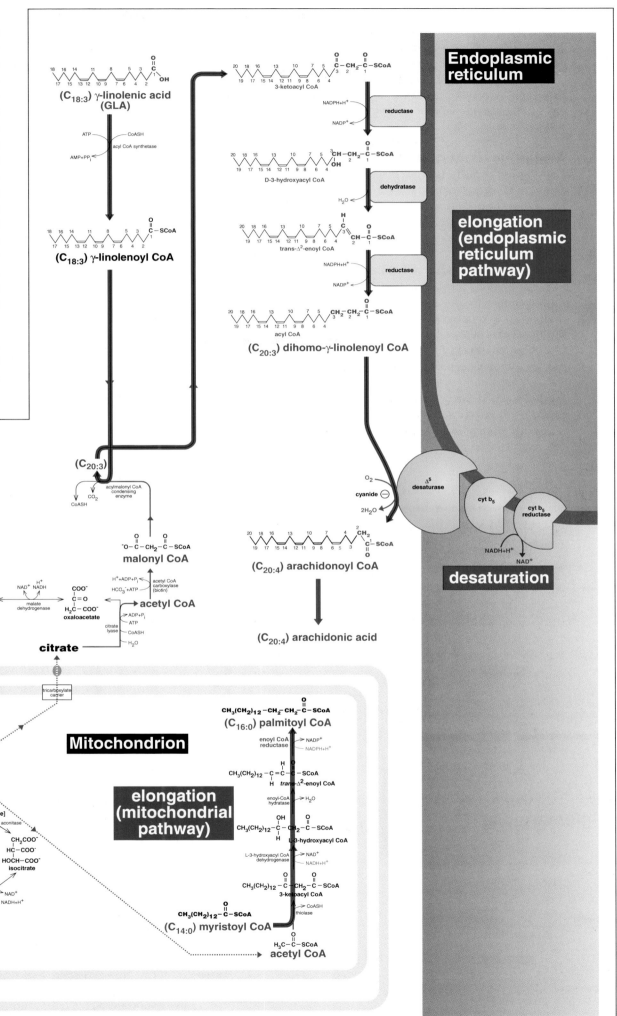

Chart 31.1 Elongation and desaturation of fatty acids.

Cholesterol, bile acids, vitamin D and the steroid hormones

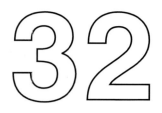

Cholesterol: friend or foe?

Despite cholesterol's notorious reputation as a major cause of cardio-vascular disease, this much maligned molecule has many useful functions. It is a major component of membranes, particularly myelin in the nervous system. Cholesterol is the precursor of the **bile salts** and of the **steroid hormones**. Intermediates involved in cholesterol biosynthesis are precursors of **ubiquinone**, **dolichol**, **vitamin D** and the **geranyl and farnesyl isoprenoid** groups, which anchor proteins to membranes.

Biosynthesis of cholesterol

Cholesterol is normally available in the diet, but it can also be synthesized from acetyl CoA derived from **glucose** or **palmitate** as shown in Chart 32.1. The enzyme controlling cholesterol synthesis is **HMG CoA reductase**, the regulation of which is complex. However, it can be inhibited by the 'statin' drugs, which are used to treat hypercholesterolaemia.

Smith–Lemli–Opitz (SLO) syndrome

Although originally classified in 1964, the chemical pathology of SLO was not determined until 1993 and was shown by Tint *et al.* to be caused by deficiency of Δ^7-dehydrocholesterol reductase (see Chart 32.1). Arguably it is thought to be the third most common inborn error of metabolism in the USA, after cystic fibrosis and phenylketonuria. The condition is characterized by multiple deformities, impaired brain development with abnormal myelination, and hypocholesterolaemia. It is thought that SLO is frequently not diagnosed, and is simply designated as 'multiple congenital abnormality syndrome of unknown aetiology'.

Another disorder of cholesterol biosynthesis is desmosterolosis but, to date, only two cases have been described. However, as analytical techniques

improve for identifying the precursors of cholesterol, it is likely that other disorders of cholesterol metabolism will be discovered.

The bile acids (salts)

Biosynthesis of the bile salts **cholate** and **chenodeoxycholate** from cholesterol is regulated by **7-α-hydroxylase** (see Chart 32.1). The bile salts are conjugated with glycine or taurine to form the glycine- or tauro-conjugates.

The steroid hormones

The principal steroid hormones are **aldosterone** (mineralocorticoid), **cortisol** (glucocorticoid), **testosterone** and **dihydrotestosterone** (androgens), and **oestradiol** (oestrogen) (see Chart 32.2). Aldosterone is synthesized in the region of the adrenal cortex called the zona glomerulosa, whereas cortisol is made in both the zona fasciculata and zona reticularis. Similarly, the sex hormones testosterone and oestradiol are synthesized *de novo* from acetyl CoA precursors or from cholesterol in the testes and ovaries respectively.

The steroid hormones are synthesized from cholesterol by pathways with a common point of control. It is thought that the translocation of cholesterol into the mitochondrion is regulated by the **St**eroid **A**cute **R**egulatory protein (**StAR**), which may be governed by the trophic hormones. (**NB:** the mitochondrial peripheral benzodiazepine receptor (PBR), which is not shown in the chart, may also be involved in cholesterol uptake.) Here **cholesterol desmolase** cleaves the side chain to form **pregnenolone**, which is the precursor of all the steroid hormones. A series of cytochrome P450-dependent reactions follow, which consume NADPH making substantial energy demands on the cell.

Chart 32.1 (opposite) Biosynthesis of cholesterol, the bile acids and vitamin D. Until recently, it was thought the reactions of cholesterol biosynthesis occurred in the cytosol and the endoplasmic reticulum. It is now known that the peroxisomes are also involved which explains the low serum cholesterol concentrations seen in peroxisomal deficiency disorders such as Zellweger syndrome.

Chart 32.2 Biosynthesis of the steroid hormones.

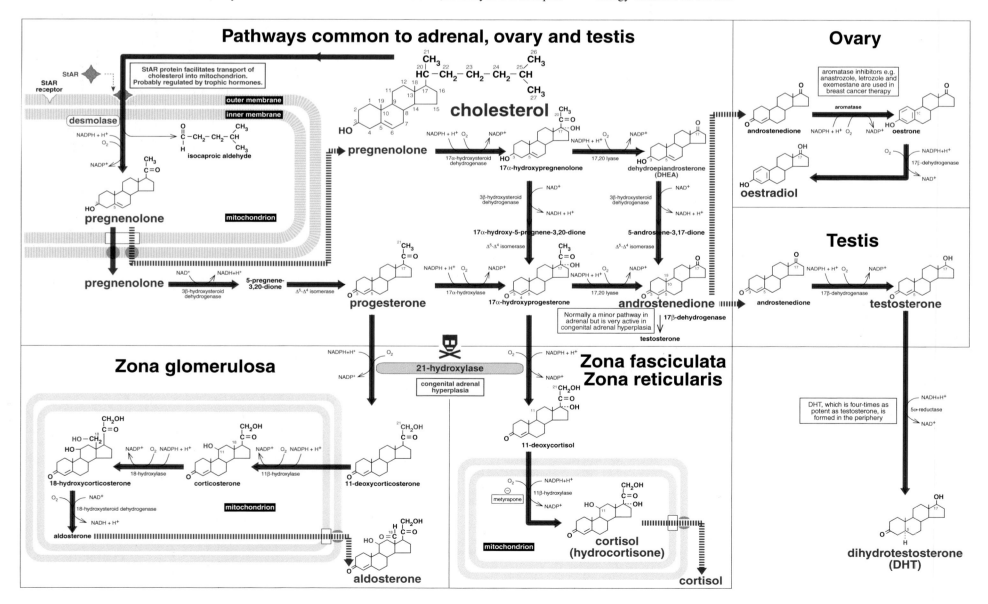

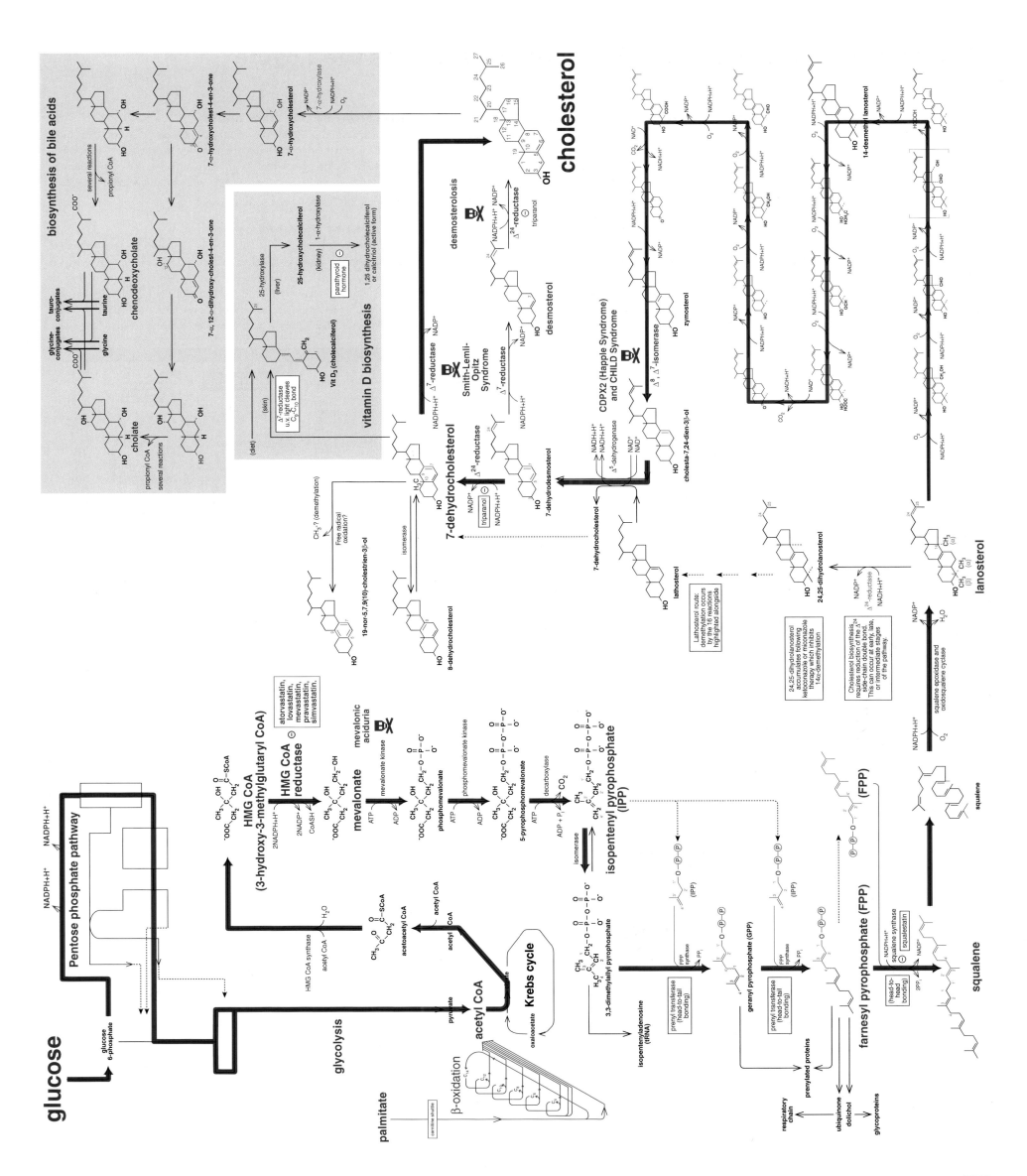

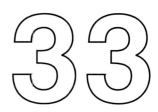

Chart 33.1 (opposite) Nitrogen, in the form of ammonium ions or glutamate, is used for urea synthesis.

A study of the other metabolic cycle elucidated by Krebs, the 'Krebs–Henseleit ornithine cycle' – popularly (but inaccurately) known as the 'urea cycle' – offers an overview of amino acid metabolism. In the fed state, any amino acids surplus to requirement for protein synthesis can be metabolized to non-nitrogenous substances such as glucose, glycogen or fatty acids, or they can be oxidized to generate ATP. On the other hand, during fasting or starvation, catabolic wasting of muscle occurs thereby yielding amino acids that are used for gluconeogenesis to maintain normoglycaemia. Because the ammonia derived from these amino acids is extremely toxic, it is converted to non-toxic **urea** for urinary excretion. Any ammonia that evades detoxification as urea can alternatively be incorporated into **glutamine** by glutamine synthetase, which has been described by Häussinger as serving as a scavenger for stray ammonium ions.

The origins of the nitrogen used for urea synthesis

In the fed state, amino acids are formed from dietary proteins by proteolytic digestion in the gastrointestinal tract. The amino acids are then absorbed into the bloodstream and may be used intact for protein synthesis. Alternatively, surplus amino acids can be metabolized to glucose, be used for fatty acid synthesis, or be catabolized to generate ATP. The amino groups are removed by transamination and deamination prior to urea synthesis in the periportal hepatocytes. The residual carbon skeletons are metabolized to the gluconeogenic precursors: pyruvate, succinyl CoA, fumarate, α-ketoglutarate, oxaloacetate or, alternatively, to the ketone bodies or their precursors (see Chapters 38 & 27, respectively).

In starvation, the circulating amino acids are derived mainly from proteolysis of muscle protein. Transamination of the amino acids, particularly the branched-chain amino acids isoleucine, valine and leucine (see Chart 33.1) occurs in the muscle in partnership with pyruvate, so that the amino acid pool in the venous blood draining from the muscle is enriched with alanine (see Chapter 36). This alanine is transported to the liver, entering via the hepatic artery, where transamination with α-ketoglutarate (α-KG) occurs to form glutamate.

Chart 33.1: Nitrogen, in the form of ammonium ions or glutamate, is used for urea synthesis

As shown in Chart 33.1, amino acids, whether of dietary or endogenous (muscle) origin, enter the pathway for urea synthesis by the **transdeamination route** or the **transamination route**.

Transdeamination route

This route consists of an initial transamination in the cytosol, followed by deamination in the mitochondrion. Initially α-**ketoglutarate** accepts an amino group from the donor amino acid to form **glutamate** in a cytosolic reaction catalysed by an **aminotransferase**. The glutamate is then transported by the glutamate carrier into the mitochondrion where it is oxidatively deaminated by **glutamate dehydrogenase** to form α-ketoglutarate and **ammonium ions**. The ammonium is incorporated into **carbamoyl phosphate**, which in turn reacts with **ornithine** to enter the urea cycle as **citrulline**.

Transamination route

Alternatively, nitrogen from the amino acids can enter the urea cycle via the transamination route, which involves two transamination reactions. Again, α-**ketoglutarate** initially accepts the amino group from the donor amino acid and once again **glutamate** is formed as described above. However, a second transamination now follows, with **oxaloacetate** accepting the amino group from glutamate to form **aspartate** in a reaction catalysed by **aspartate aminotransferase (AST)**. This aspartate now carries the second amino group into the urea cycle by condensing with **citrulline** to form **argininosuccinate**. Argininosuccinate is then cleaved to form **fumarate** and **arginine**. Finally, arginine is hydrolysed to **ornithine** and **urea**, and ornithine is regenerated for another rotation of the cycle.

Regulation of the urea cycle

The condensation of ammonia with bicarbonate to form carbamoyl phosphate is catalysed by **carbamoyl phosphate synthetase (CPS)**, which is only active in the presence of its allosteric effector, **N-acetylglutamate (NAG)**. NAG is synthesized from acetyl CoA and glutamate by *N*-acetylglutamate synthase.

Disorders of the urea cycle

The most common urea cycle disorder is ornithine transcarbamoylase (OTC) deficiency, which is X-linked. Affected boys develop severe hyperammonaemia, which often leads to early death. However, in heterozygous girls, the condition can vary from being undetectable to a severity equal to that in boys. In this condition, carbamoyl phosphate accumulates and passes into the cytosol where it reacts with aspartate to form carbamoyl aspartate.

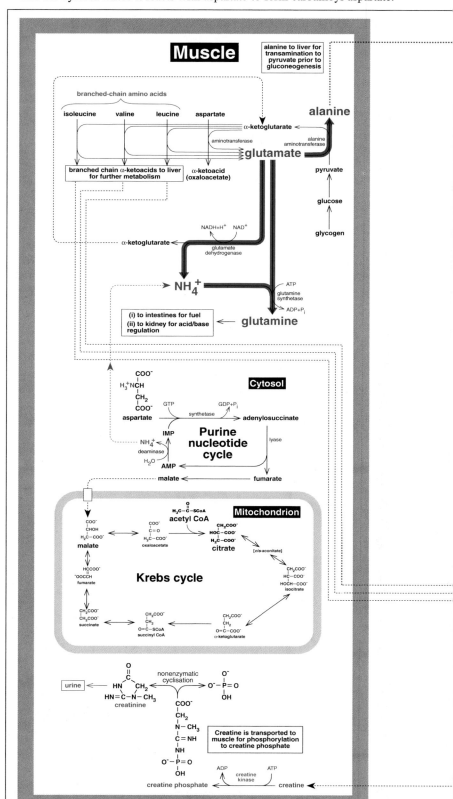

This is metabolized to form orotate by the reactions described for pyrimidine synthesis in Chapter 44. Detection of orotic acid (orotic aciduria) in urine is used to diagnose OTC deficiency.

OTC deficiency and gene therapy

There was considerable optimism that OTC deficiency would be a model candidate for liver-directed gene therapy. Unfortunately, a pilot study on 17 subjects with partial OTC deficiency using an adenoviral vector was very disappointing. There was very little gene transfer and when subject 18 suffered lethal complications, the trial was stopped.

Creatine and creatinine

The main function of the ornithine cycle is to produce urea. However, as shown in the chart, a small but significant quantity of arginine is diverted to form creatine. This is phosphorylated by creatine kinase to produce **creatine phosphate**, which is the phosphagen used to generate ATP during short bursts of intensive exercise. Approximately 2% of the body pool of creatine phosphate spontaneously cyclizes each day and is excreted in the urine as creatinine.

The purine nucleotide cycle

The purine nucleotide cycle described by Lowenstein, although present in many types of tissues, is particularly active in muscle. During vigorous exercise in rats, the blood concentration of ammonium ions can increase five-fold. This ammonium is thought to be derived from aspartate via the purine nucleotide cycle. This cycle is mentioned in Chapter 24.

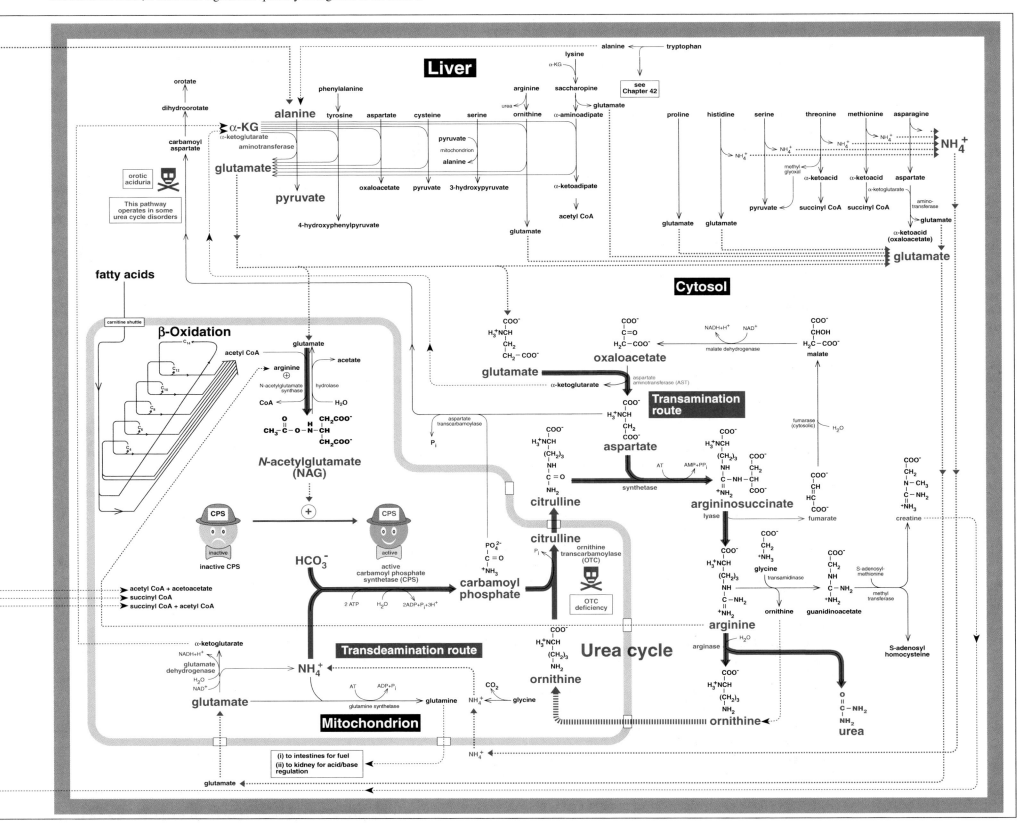

Metabolic channelling: enzymes are organized to enable channelling of metabolic intermediates

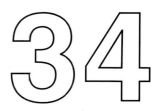

Diagram 34.3 (opposite) Partial metabolic channelling in the urea cycle. Channelling is interrupted when ornithine and citrulline diffuse across the intermembrane space. During this stage of the journey, the molecules are free to equilibrate with other molecules in the intermembrane space and so metabolic channelling does not occur.

Diagram 34.1 Enzymes associating with citrate synthase. A schematic representation of how the enzymes and carrier proteins involved in the reactions adjacent to citrate synthase might be organized to allow metabolic channelling.

Diagram 34.2 Experimental approach to demonstrate metabolic channelling by radioisotope dilution. 34.2(a) This represents a pathway from substrate A, which is metabolized via intermediates B and C to product D. If A is radioactive, then the specific radioactivity of intermediates B and C and product D will all be the same. **34.2(b)** If a 200-fold excess of non-radioactive C is added, then provided substrate channelling does not occur, radioactive C will equilibrate with non-radioactive C and the specific radioactivity of product D will be diluted 200-fold. **34.2(c)** If the experiment in **34.2(b)** is repeated but metabolic channelling does occur, then the 200-fold excess of non-radioactive C will not equilibrate with radioactive C and the specific radioactivity of D will be the same as A.

Metabolic intermediates are channelled from enzyme to enzyme

When I was a student it was rather assumed that the cell was 'a bag of enzymes' and that their substrates were randomly moving throughout the cytoplasm until a chance collision brought enzyme and substrate together enabling the reaction to proceed. It was imagined that the product of this reaction would diffuse through the aqueous environment until a chance encounter with the next enzyme and substrate occurred to form the next product, and so on through to the end of the metabolic pathway. However, this simplistic idea is very inefficient and P.A. Srere introduced the hypothesis of **metabolic channelling**. This concept proposes that the products of an enzyme reaction are passed directly from the enzyme to the next enzyme in the metabolic sequence. This was defined by Srere as follows:

> '*Metabolic channelling of an intermediate can be defined as the passage of a common intermediate between two enzymes. The intermediate is localised and is out of equilibrium with the bulk solution.*'

Experimental evidence supporting 'metabolic channelling'
Co-precipitation of enzymes

One of several experimental approaches that provides compelling evidence in support of metabolic channelling is provided by the tendency of enzymes that are sequential in a metabolic pathway to associate and co-precipitate when studied under certain conditions. Although enzymes when studied in dilute solution *in vitro* are free to diffuse in search of their substrates, this is not the case *in vivo*. For example, the proportion of soluble protein in the mitochondrial matrix is approximately 500 mg/ml of water. This water is approximately 50% water of hydration leaving just 50% free. These conditions can be simulated *in vitro* by adding to an enzyme preparation a volume-excluder, such as polyethyleneglycol, that removes water causing the enzymes to crowd together. This results in enzymes that are next to each other in a metabolic sequence to associate and co-precipitate. For example the mitochondrial enzyme **citrate synthase** has been shown to bind to and co-precipitate with **pyruvate carboxylase**, the **pyruvate carrier**, **pyruvate dehydrogenase** and the **tricarboxylate transporter**. As shown in Diagram 34.1, these enzymes and carrier proteins are sequential in the pathways for pyruvate metabolism in mitochondria. Moreover, the binding is specific; for example, **citrate synthase** binds to the **mitochondrial** isoform of **malate dehydrogenase** but not to the **cytosolic** isoform of this enzyme.

Isotope dilution studies

Further evidence for metabolic channelling is provided by radioisotope dilution studies. Diagram 34.2a represents a metabolic pathway in which a radiolabelled substrate A is metabolized via intermediates B and C to product D. If the substrates and their enzymes are free to diffuse in solution **(i.e. if there is no channelling of the metabolites)**, then at steady state the specific activity of B, C and D will be the same as A. If now as shown in

Diagram 34.2b, a 200-fold excess of non-radioactive C is added, then **in the absence of channelling**, the specific radioactivity of C and product D will be diluted 200-fold, i.e. to 0.5% of the original value.

However, as represented metaphorically in Diagram 34.2c, if the metabolites and their enzymes are prevented from freely diffusing in the surrounding solution, i.e. the intermediates are passed from enzyme to enzyme and **metabolite channelling is occurring**, then addition of a 200-fold excess of non-radioactive C will not dilute the specific radioactivity of the product D. Instead, D is formed from the channelled radioactive C rather than from the pool of non-radioactive C in the bulk solution.

Metabolic channelling in the urea cycle

Experiments using radioisotope dilution studies suggest that metabolic channelling occurs in the urea cycle, albeit incompletely (see Diagram 34.3). An experiment used **α-toxin** to make pores in the plasma membrane of hepatocytes. The hepatocytes were incubated in a physiological medium with ¹⁴**C-labelled** HCO_3^-, **aspartate** and **ammonium chloride** as carbon and nitrogen sources plus other essential compounds. The ¹⁴C label appeared in **urea** as would be anticipated. When a 200-fold excess of **non-radioactive arginine** was added, there was no decrease in the specific radioactivity of the urea formed. This suggests that metabolic channelling occurs between the **lyase** and **arginase** enzymes. However, when a 200-fold excess of **non-radioactive citrulline** was added, the specific radioactivity of the urea formed was reduced. This is because **citrulline** is formed by enzymes on the mitochondrial inner membrane and must diffuse across the intermembrane space to **argininosuccinate synthetase**, which is located on the outer side of the outer mitochondrial membrane. While ¹⁴C-citrulline is diffusing across the intermembrane space metabolic channelling is not occurring and the radiolabelled citrulline is diluted with the added non-radioactive citrulline.

Reference

Cohen N.S., Cheung C.W. & Raijman L. (1996) The urea cycle. In *Channelling in Intermediary Metabolism* (L. Agius & H.S.A. Sherratt, eds), 183–99. Portland Press, London and Miami.

Diagram 34.2

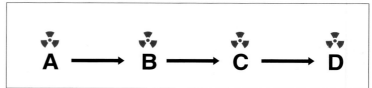

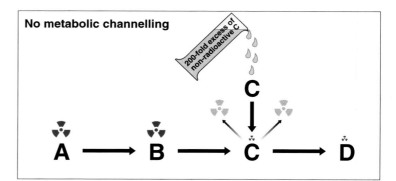

No metabolic channelling

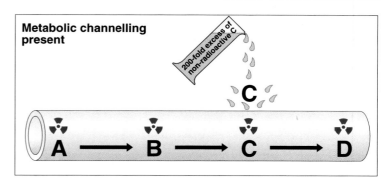

Metabolic channelling present

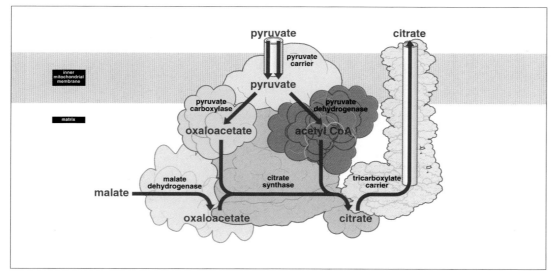

Diagram 34.1

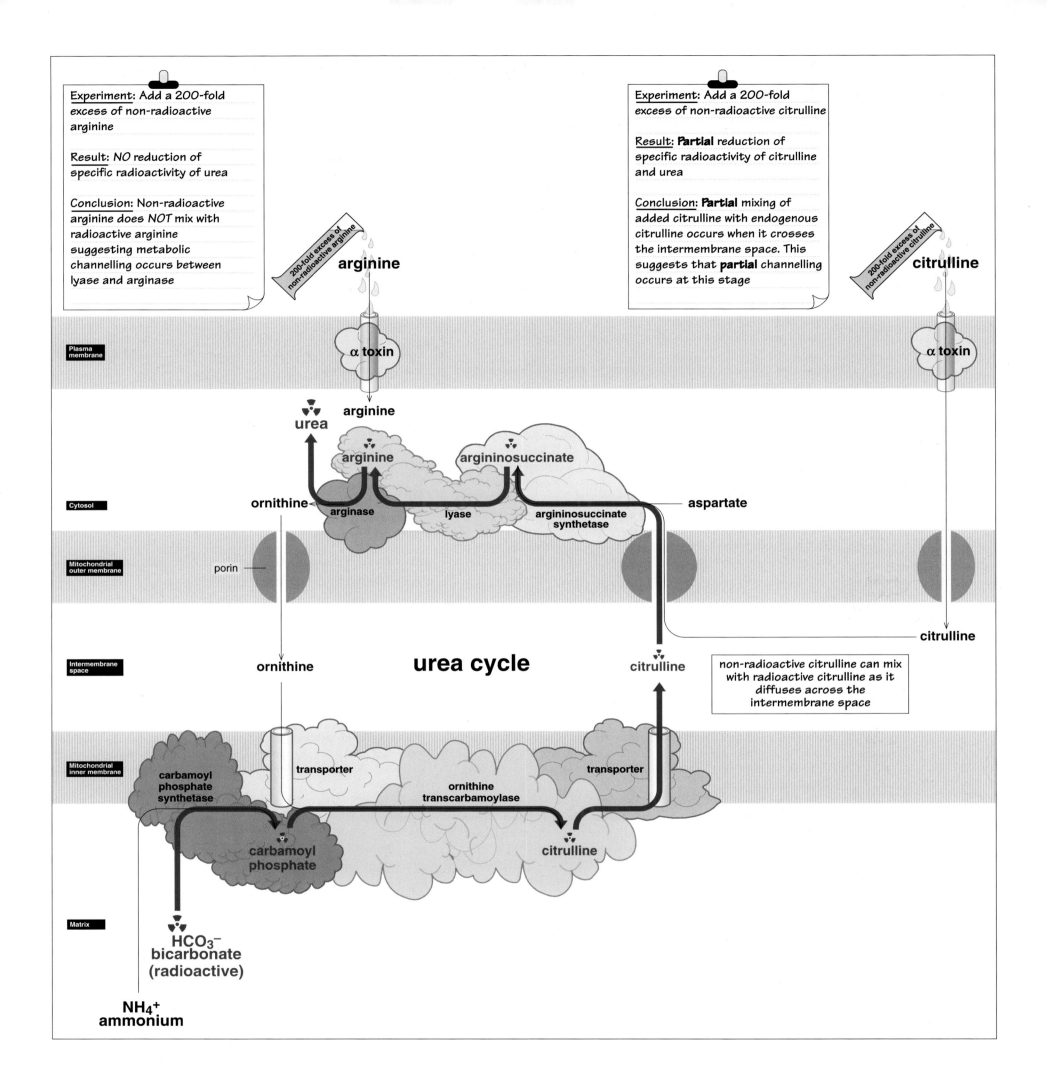

Biosynthesis of the non-essential amino acids

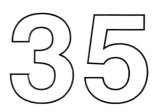

Chart 35.1 (opposite)
Biosynthesis of the non-essential amino acids.

Whereas plants and some bacteria are capable of synthesizing all of the amino acids necessary for the formation of cellular proteins and other vital molecules, this is not the case in mammals. Mammals, including humans, can synthesize only 11 of these amino acids, namely tyrosine, aspartate, asparagine, alanine, serine, glycine, cysteine, glutamate, glutamine, proline and arginine. These are known as the **non-essential amino acids**, and their biosynthesis is shown in Chart 35.1. The other nine amino acids – phenylalanine, threonine, methionine, lysine, tryptophan, leucine, isoleucine, valine and histidine – cannot be synthesized. They are known as the **essential amino acids**.

Tyrosine

Biosynthesis of tyrosine. Tyrosine is formed from the essential amino acid phenylalanine in the presence of phenylalanine monooxygenase.

Uses. Tyrosine is a precursor in the synthesis of adrenaline, noradrenaline, thyroxine and the pigment, melanin.

Serine, glycine and cysteine

These amino acids are made from intermediates formed by glycolysis.

Biosynthesis of serine. Serine is synthesized by a pathway commonly known as 'the phosphorylated pathway'. First, 3-phosphoglycerate is oxidized to 3-phosphohydroxypyruvate, which is then transaminated to 3-phosphoserine. Finally, hydrolysis by a specific phosphatase yields serine. This phosphoserine phosphatase is inhibited by serine providing feedback regulation of the pathway. **NB:** The so-called 'non-phosphorylated pathway' for serine metabolism is important in the gluconeogenic state (see Chapter 38).

Uses. Serine is a component of the phospholipid, phosphatidylserine. Also, serine is a very important source of '1-carbon' precursors for biosynthesis (see Chapters 43 & 44).

Biosynthesis of glycine. Glycine can be formed by two routes, both of which involve serine. Glycine is formed from serine by a reversible reaction catalysed by **serine hydroxymethyltransferase**, which is a pyridoxal phosphate-dependent enzyme existing as both cytosolic and mitochondrial isoforms. This enzyme uses the coenzyme tetrahydrofolate (THF), which is formed by reduction of the vitamin folic acid (see Chapter 43). It accepts a 1-carbon fragment from serine to form N^5,N^{10}-methylene tetrahydrofolate, and glycine is formed.

An alternative route for glycine synthesis uses CO_2 and NH_4^+ in a reaction catalysed by the mitochondrial enzyme **glycine synthase** (also known as the glycine cleavage enzyme when working in the reverse direction (see Chapter 37). The second carbon atom is derived from N^5,N^{10}-methylene THF obtained from serine in the previously mentioned reaction catalysed by serine hydroxymethyltransferase.

Uses. The demand for **glycine** by the body is considerable, and it has been estimated that the requirement for endogenous synthesis of glycine is between 10 and 50 times the dietary intake. Apart from its contribution to cellular proteins, glycine is required for the synthesis of purines, collagen, porphyrins, creatine and glutathione and conjugation with bile salts. Glycine can also be conjugated with certain drugs and toxic substances to facilitate their excretion in the urine. Finally, glycine is made by mitochondria in brain cells, where it acts as an inhibitory neurotransmitter. Hypotheses have implicated a deficiency of serine -hydroxymethyltransferase with schizophrenia.

Biosynthesis of cysteine. Cysteine can be formed from serine provided that the essential amino acid methionine is available to donate a sulphur atom. When there is a metabolic demand for cysteine, homocysteine condenses with serine to yield cystathionine in a reaction catalysed by cystathionine synthase. Cystathionine is then cleaved by cystathionase to release cysteine.

Uses. Cysteine is a component of the tripeptide glutathione (γ-glutamylcysteinylglycine).

Aspartate and asparagine

Biosynthesis of aspartate. Aspartate is readily formed by the transamination of oxaloacetate by glutamate in the presence of aspartate aminotransferase (AST).

Uses. Aspartate is an amino donor in urea synthesis, and in both pyrimidine and purine synthesis.

Biosynthesis of asparagine. Asparagine is synthesized by amide transfer from glutamine in the presence of asparagine synthetase.

Uses. Asparagine is incorporated into cellular proteins but appears to have no other role in mammals.

Glutamate, glutamine, proline and arginine

These amino acids are formed from the Krebs cycle intermediate α-ketoglutarate.

Biosynthesis of glutamate. Glutamate is formed by the reductive amination of α-ketoglutarate by glutamate dehydrogenase.

Biosynthesis of glutamine. Glutamine is formed from glutamate and NH_4^+ in an ATP-requiring reaction catalysed by glutamine synthetase (see Chapters 33 & 36).

Uses. Glutamine is a very important source of nitrogen for purine and pyrimidine (and hence nucleic acid) synthesis (see Chapters 43 & 44). Glutamine also is important in regulating pH in acidotic conditions.

Biosynthesis of proline. In the presence of pyrroline 5-carboxylate synthetase, glutamate is converted to glutamate γ-semialdehyde, which spontaneously cyclizes to pyrroline 5-carboxylate. This can then be reduced to proline.

Biosynthesis of arginine. Pyrroline 5-carboxylate is in equilibrium with glutamate γ-semialdehyde, which can be transaminated by ornithine transaminase to yield ornithine. Ornithine can then enter the urea cycle and so form arginine (see Chapter 33).

Uses. Arginine is an intermediate in the urea cycle and is the precursor of creatine. It is also the source of the vasodilator nitric oxide.

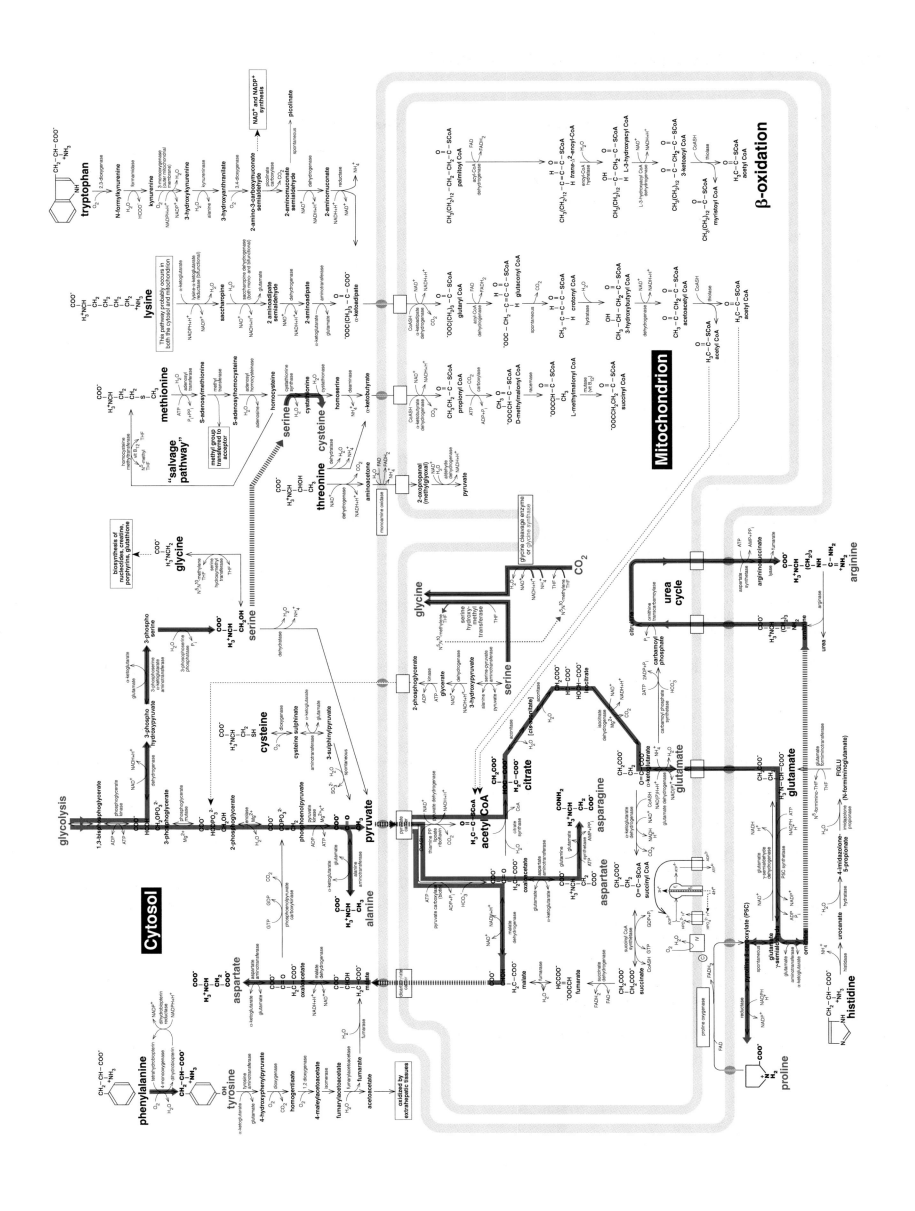

Catabolism of amino acids I

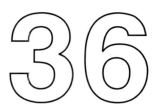

36

Chart 36.1 (opposite) Formation of alanine and glutamine by muscle.

Proteins, whether of dietary origin in the fed state or derived from muscle protein in starvation, can be degraded to amino acids for direct oxidation as a respiratory fuel with the generation of ATP. However, it is also possible that, in the fed state, amino acids may first be converted to glycogen or triacylglycerol for fuel storage prior to energy metabolism. Alternatively, in starvation, certain glucogenic amino acids are initially converted in muscle to alanine, which is subsequently converted by the liver to glucose to provide fuel for the brain and red blood cells. Finally, the ketogenic amino acids form the ketone bodies, which are a valuable fuel for the brain in starvation.

The catabolism of aspartate and the branched-chain amino acids (BCAAs) will be emphasized here, and catabolism of the remaining amino acids will be described in Chapter 37.

Dietary protein as a source of energy in the fed state

Protein is digested in the gastrointestinal tract to release its 20 constituent amino acids. If they are surplus to the body's requirement for incorporation into proteins or other essential molecules derived from amino acids, they may be metabolized to glycogen or fat (see Chapters 38 & 39) and subsequently used for energy metabolism. Alternatively, they can be oxidized directly as a metabolic fuel. However, different tissues have different abilities to catabolize the various amino acids.

Metabolism of muscle protein during starvation or prolonged exercise

In the fed state, muscle uses glucose and fatty acids for energy metabolism. However, during fasting, starvation or prolonged exercise, protein from muscle plays an important role in glucose homeostasis. For example, during an overnight fast the hepatic glycogen reserves can be depleted and life-threatening hypoglycaemia must be prevented. Remember that fat cannot be converted to glucose (see Chapter 14), apart from the glycerol derived from triacylglycerol metabolism. Consequently, muscle tissue remains as the only glucogenic source and must be 'sacrificed' to maintain blood glucose concentrations and thus ensure a vital supply of energy for the red blood cells and the brain.

During starvation, muscle protein must first be broken down into its constituent amino acids, but the details of intracellular proteolysis are still not fully understood. It was once thought that, following proteolysis, all of the different amino acids were released from the muscle into the blood in proportion to their composition in muscle proteins. Research has shown that this idea is more complicated than originally supposed. During fasting, the blood draining from muscle is especially enriched with alanine and glutamine, which can each constitute up to 30% of the total amino acids released

by muscle, a proportion greatly in excess of their relative abundance in muscle proteins. Alanine released from muscle is taken up by the liver in a process known as the **glucose alanine cycle**. Glutamine is not taken up by the liver, but is used by the intestines as a fuel and by the kidney for gluconeogenesis and pH homeostasis.

Catabolism of the branched-chain amino acids (BCAAs)

The oxidation of the branched-chain amino acids (leucine, isoleucine and valine) is shown in Chart 36.1. The branched-chain α-ketoacid dehydrogenase (BCKADH) resembles pyruvate dehydrogenase. Moreover, the oxidation of the acyl CoA derivatives formed by this reaction has many similarities with the β-oxidation of fatty acids, which is included in Chart 36.1 for the purpose of comparison. **NB:** Not all tissues can oxidize the BCAAs. Whereas muscle has BCAA aminotransferase activity, liver lacks this enzyme. However, liver has BCKADH activity and can oxidize the branched-chain ketoacids.

It should be noted that, in starvation and diabetes, the activity of muscle BCKADH is increased up to five-fold, thereby promoting oxidation of the BCAAs in muscle.

Chart 36.1: Formation of alanine and glutamine by muscle
Alanine and the glucose alanine cycle
The glucose alanine cycle was proposed by Felig, who demonstrated increased production of alanine by muscle during starvation. The BCAAs are the major donors of amino groups for alanine synthesis. Pyruvate, for transamination to alanine, can be formed from isoleucine and valine (via succinyl CoA), from certain other amino acids (e.g. aspartate) or, alternatively, from glycolysis. The alanine so formed is exported from muscle and is transported via the hepatic artery to the liver, where it is used for gluconeogenesis (see Diagram 36.1).

Glutamine
Glutamine is the most abundant amino acid in the blood. As shown in Chart 36.1 (and Chart 33.1), BCAAs are major donors of the amino groups used to form glutamate, which is further aminated by glutamine synthetase to form glutamine.

The ketogenic amino acids leucine and isoleucine as an energy source
As shown in Chart 36.1, the entire carbon skeleton of leucine and carbon fragments from isoleucine are converted to acetoacetate or to acetyl CoA, which can be converted into acetoacetate in the liver (see Chapter 27). The ketone bodies can then be oxidized as a respiratory fuel by extrahepatic tissues, as described in Chapter 28.

Diagram 36.1
Formation of alanine from muscle protein. In starvation, the amino acids derived from muscle protein are degraded to ketoacids. Some of the carbon skeletons from these ketoacids enter Krebs cycle and are metabolized via phosphoenolpyruvate carboxykinase (PEPCK) and pyruvate kinase (PK) to pyruvate. Alanine amino-transferase (ALT) is very active in muscle and so much of the pyruvate produced is transaminated to alanine which leaves the muscle and is transported in the blood to the liver.
Gluconeogenesis from alanine in the liver. In the liver, alanine is reconverted to pyruvate which is used for gluconeogenesis. **NB:** Pyruvate kinase in the liver is inhibited in the gluconeogenic state both by protein kinase A phosphorylation, and directly by alanine (see Chapter 23). This prevents the futile recycling of pyruvate which would otherwise happen. The glucose formed can be used for energy metabolism, especially by the brain and red blood cells.

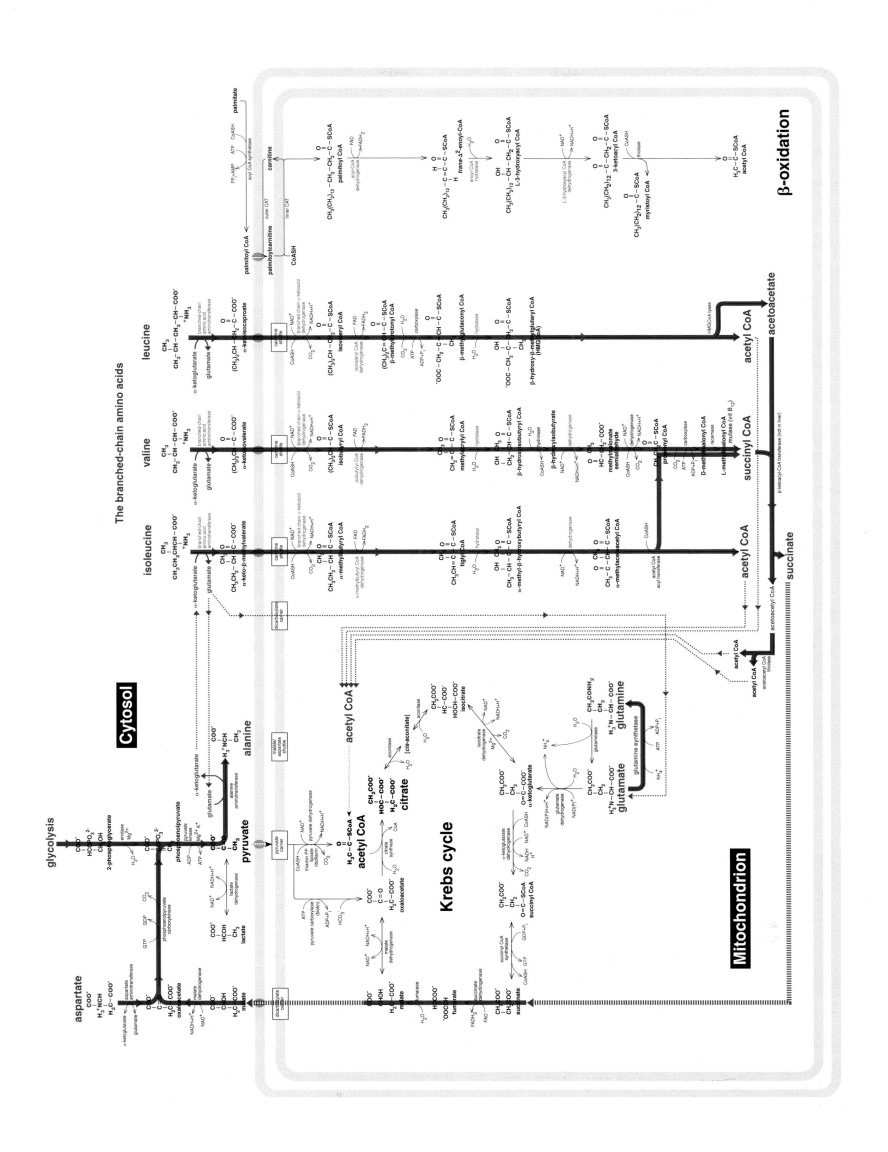

Catabolism of amino acids II

37

Alanine. Alanine is in equilibrium with pyruvate, which is oxidatively decarboxylated to CO_2 and acetyl CoA. The latter can then be oxidized in Krebs cycle.

Glycine. Although there are several possible routes for glycine catabolism, the mitochondrial 'glycine cleavage system' is probably the most important in mammals. This enzyme complex is loosely bound to the mitochondrial inner membrane and has several similarities to the pyruvate dehydrogenase complex. It oxidatively decarboxylates glycine to carbon dioxide and N^5,N^{10}-methylene-tetrahydrofolate (N^5,N^{10}-THF).

Serine. When needed as a respiratory fuel, serine undergoes deamination by serine dehydratase to form pyruvate, as shown in Chart 37.1.

Threonine. The most important route for the catabolism of threonine in mammals is the 'aminoacetone pathway'. Threonine dehydrogenase forms the unstable intermediate α-amino-β-ketobutyrate, which is spontaneously decarboxylated to aminoacetone for further catabolism to pyruvate.
It is possible that threonine is also deaminated by serine dehydratase and by a specific threonine dehydratase to form α-ketobutyrate. This could then be metabolized to succinyl CoA, as outlined for methionine metabolism.

Cysteine. There are several possible pathways for cysteine degradation but the most important in mammals is oxidation by cysteine dioxygenase to cysteine sulphinate. This is then transaminated to form 3-sulphinylpyruvate (also known as β-mercaptopyruvate or thiopyruvate), which is converted to pyruvate in a spontaneous reaction.

Methionine. Methionine is activated in an ATP-dependent reaction to form S-adenosylmethionine (SAM), which is the major carrier of methyl groups, beating THF into second place as a donor in biosynthetic methylations. For example, SAM is used in the methylation of noradrenaline to adrenaline by noradrenaline N-methyltransferase. Consequently, the original methionine molecule is demethylated to form S-adenosyl homocysteine, then the adenosyl group is removed to homocysteine. This intermediate can be metabolized in two ways:
1 It can be recycled to methionine in a salvage pathway where the methyl donor is N^5-methyl-THF, using a vitamin B_{12}-dependent reaction catalysed by homocysteine methyltransferase. This is an important pathway which helps to conserve this essential amino acid.
2 It can be degraded to succinyl CoA, which can be further metabolized to pyruvate for energy metabolism.

Lysine. Lysine is unusual in that it cannot be formed from its corresponding α-ketoacid, α-keto-ε-aminocaproic acid, which cyclizes to form Δ^1-piperidine-2-carboxylic acid. Degradation of lysine occurs via saccharopine, a compound in which lysine and α-ketoglutarate are bonded as a secondary amine formed with the carbonyl group of α-ketoglutarate and the ε-amino group of lysine. Following two further dehydrogenase reactions, α-ketoadipate is formed by transamination. This enters the mitochondrion and is oxidized by a pathway with many similarities to the β-oxidation pathway. Acetoacetyl CoA is formed, thus lysine is classified as a ketogenic amino acid (see Chapter 27).

Tryptophan. Although tryptophan can be oxidized as a respiratory fuel, it is also an important precursor for the synthesis of NAD^+ and $NADP^+$ (see Chapter 42). The regulatory mechanisms involved in the first step of tryptophan catabolism catalysed by tryptophan dioxygenase (also known as tryptophan pyrrolase) have been studied extensively. It is known that the dioxygenase is induced by glucocorticoids, which increase transcription of DNA. Furthermore, glucagon (via cyclic adenosine monophosphate, cAMP) increases the synthesis of dioxygenase by enhancing the translation of mRNA. Hence in starvation, the combined effects of these hormones will promote the oxidation of tryptophan released from muscle protein.

During the catabolism of tryptophan, the amino group is retained in the first three intermediates formed. The amino group in the form of alanine is then hydrolytically cleaved from 3-hydroxykynurenine by kynureninase. This alanine molecule can then be transaminated to pyruvate, thus qualifying tryptophan as a glucogenic amino acid. The other product of kynureninase is 3-hydroxyanthranilate, which is degraded to α-ketoadipate. This is oxidized by a pathway which is similar to β-oxidation to form acetoacetyl CoA. Hence tryptophan is both a ketogenic and a glucogenic amino acid.

Glutamate. This readily enters Krebs cycle following oxidative deamination by glutamate dehydrogenase as α-ketoglutarate. However, for complete oxidation its metabolites must temporarily leave the cycle for conversion to pyruvate. This can then be oxidized to acetyl CoA, which enters Krebs cycle for energy metabolism, generating ATP.

Histidine. Histidine is metabolized to glutamate by a pathway which involves the elimination of a 1-carbon group. In this reaction, the formimino group (–CH=NH) is transferred from N-formiminoglutamate (FIGLU) to THF, yielding N^5-formimino-THF and glutamate.

Arginine. This amino acid is a constituent of proteins as well as being an intermediate in the urea cycle. Arginine is cleaved by arginase to liberate urea, and ornithine is formed. Ornithine is transaminated by ornithine aminotransferase to form glutamate γ-semialdehyde. The semialdehyde is then oxidized by glutamate γ-semialdehyde dehydrogenase to form glutamate.

Proline. The catabolism of proline to glutamate differs from its biosynthetic pathway. Proline is oxidized by the mitochondrial enzyme proline oxygenase, to form pyrroline 5-carboxylate. This is probably an FAD-dependent enzyme, located in the inner mitochondrial membrane, which can donate electrons directly to cytochrome c in the electron transport chain.

Chart 37.1 (opposite)
Catabolism of amino acids.

Chart 37.2 If amino acids are to be used as a respiratory fuel it is obligatory that their carbon skeletons are converted to acetyl CoA, which must then enter Krebs cycle for oxidation, producing ATP as described in Chapter 6. **NB:** The simple entry of the carbon skeletons into Krebs cycle as 'dicarboxylic acids' (α-ketoglutarate, succinate, fumarate or oxaloacetate) does not ensure their complete oxidation for energy metabolism.

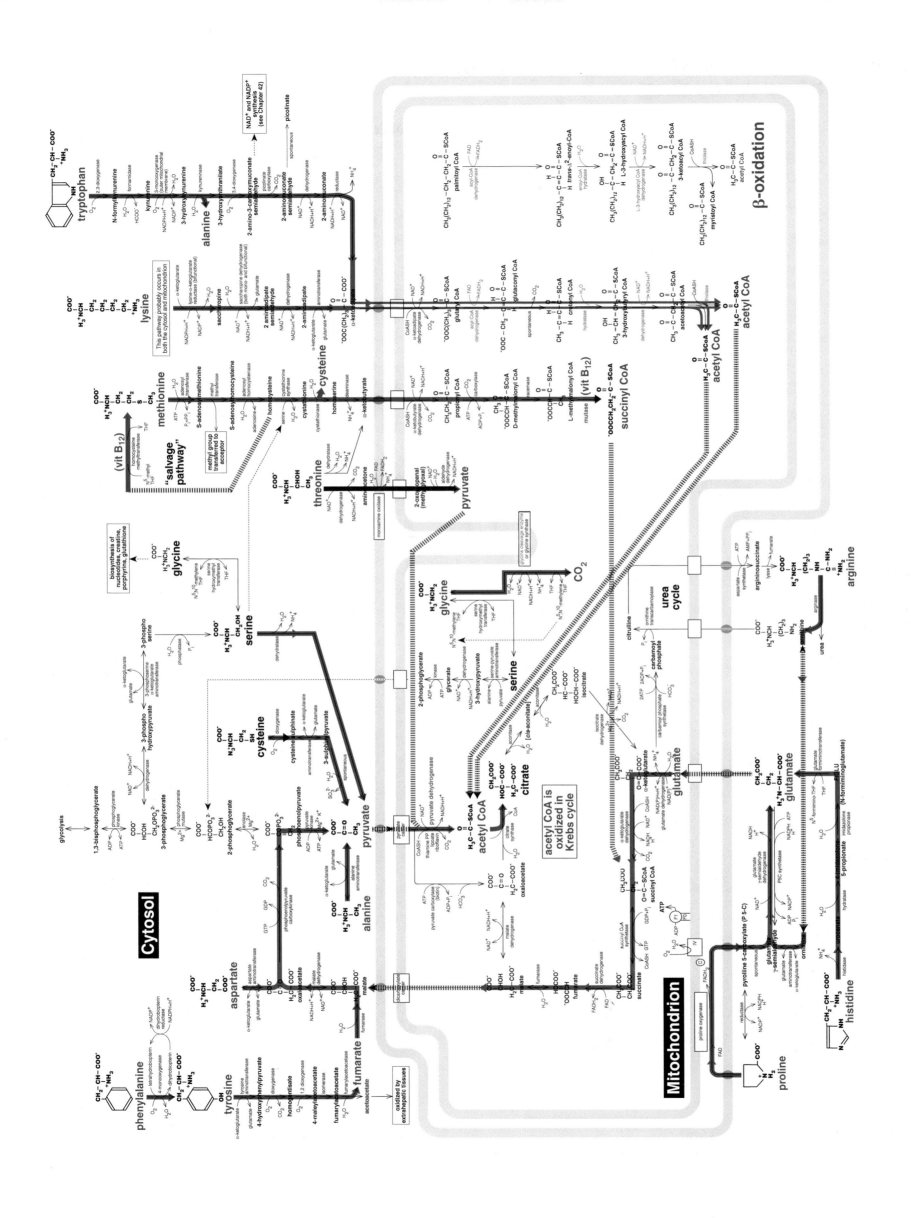

Metabolism of amino acids to glucose in starvation and during the period immediately after refeeding

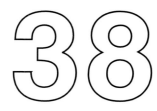

Chart 38.1 (opposite) Gluconeogenesis from amino acids.

Diagram 38.1 Intermediary metabolism in the early fed state. β-Oxidation of fatty acids continues in the early fed state. The liver continues in ketogenic and gluconeogenic modes, using lactate (from muscle) and dietary amino acids as gluconeogenic substrates. Muscle uses fatty acids and ketone bodies as respiratory fuels. Also, glycolysis is active in muscle but, since pyruvate dehydrogenase is inactive, lactate is formed.

In liver, the switch from gluconeogenic mode to glycolytic mode in the early fed state is a slow process

During starvation, when the glycogen reserves have been exhausted, muscle proteins are degraded to amino acids and used by the liver for gluconeogenesis to maintain the supply of glucose, which is vital for the brain. The important role of alanine as a gluconeogenic precursor is described in Chapter 36.

Following refeeding after a period of starvation, the liver does not switch instantaneously from gluconeogenic to glycolytic mode even though it receives a large glucose load from the intestines. In the early fed state the effects of the gluconeogenic and lipolytic hormones linger, and β-oxidation of fatty acids continues. Consequently, large quantities of acetyl CoA are produced, which inhibit pyruvate dehydrogenase, thereby favouring gluconeogenesis in the liver. Under these conditions, the amino acids derived from the gastrointestinal digestion of dietary protein can be used for gluconeogenesis, as shown in Chart 38.1 and described below.

Starvation

In starvation, hepatic gluconeogenesis is active under the hormonal influence of glucagon, cortisol and adrenocorticotropic hormone (ACTH) (see Chapter 23). Glycolysis in the liver is inhibited because glucagon, through cyclic AMP-dependent protein kinase, causes the phosphorylation of hepatic pyruvate kinase, thereby causing inhibition. Moreover, the phosphorylation of hepatic pyruvate kinase is potentiated by its allosteric effector **alanine** (which is abundant in starvation), which therefore further enhances the inhibition of pyruvate kinase.

The role of acetyl CoA in promoting gluconeogenesis in starvation

During starvation, β-oxidation from fatty acids is very active in the liver, and large quantities of acetyl CoA are formed. The accumulated acetyl CoA inhibits pyruvate dehydrogenase and stimulates pyruvate carboxylase. This means that pyruvate (derived from alanine) does not enter Krebs cycle as acetyl CoA, but is instead carboxylated by pyruvate carboxylase to oxaloacetate for metabolism to phosphoenolpyruvate and thence to glucose via gluconeogenesis.

The early fed state
Fate of the glucogenic amino acids

During refeeding after a period of starvation, the liver remains in the gluconeogenic mode for a few hours. Consequently, the glucogenic amino acids derived from dietary protein are metabolized to **2-phosphoglycerate**, which is their common precursor for gluconeogenesis (see Chart 38.1 and Diagram 38.1).

NB: Evidence suggests that gluconeogenesis from serine originates in the mitochondrion. However, the mitochondrial carriers needed for the route shown, in particular the 2-phosphoglycerate carrier, have not been characterized.

In any event, 2-phosphoglycerate is metabolized to glucose 6-phosphate, which can be used to synthesize glycogen or glucose. The amino nitrogen derived from the amino acids is detoxified as urea.

Dietary glucose is converted by muscle to lactate prior to glycogen synthesis

It is emphasized that, in the early fed state, glucose cannot be used by the liver for glycolysis. Instead, high concentrations of glucose promote hepatic glycogen synthesis. Alternatively, in the presence of insulin, glucose enters the muscle cells where it undergoes glycolysis to lactate (see Diagram 38.1). Remember that β-oxidation of fatty acids is active and produces an abundance of acetyl CoA, which inhibits muscle pyruvate dehydrogenase. This means that lactate is formed even though conditions are aerobic. The lactate is then transported to the liver, which can convert it to glycogen or glucose.

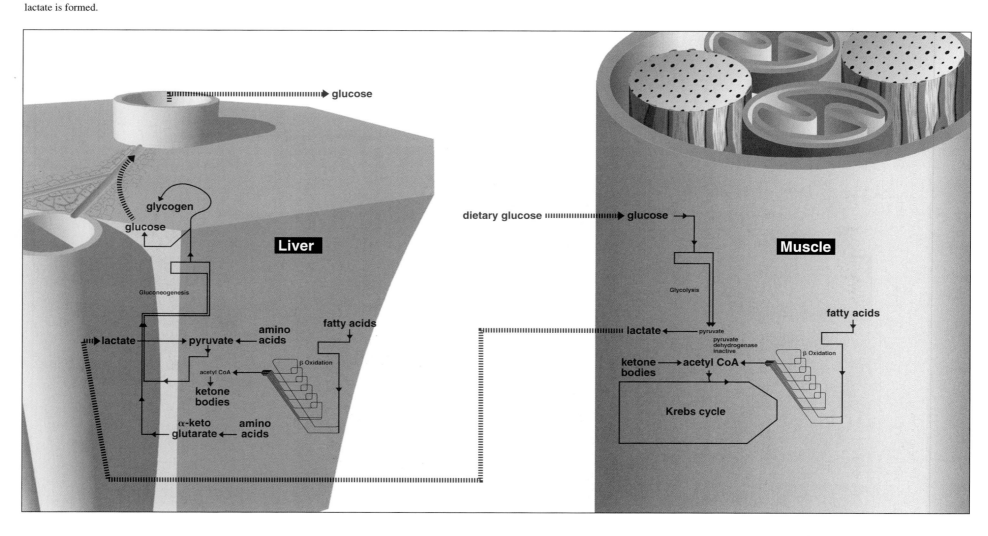

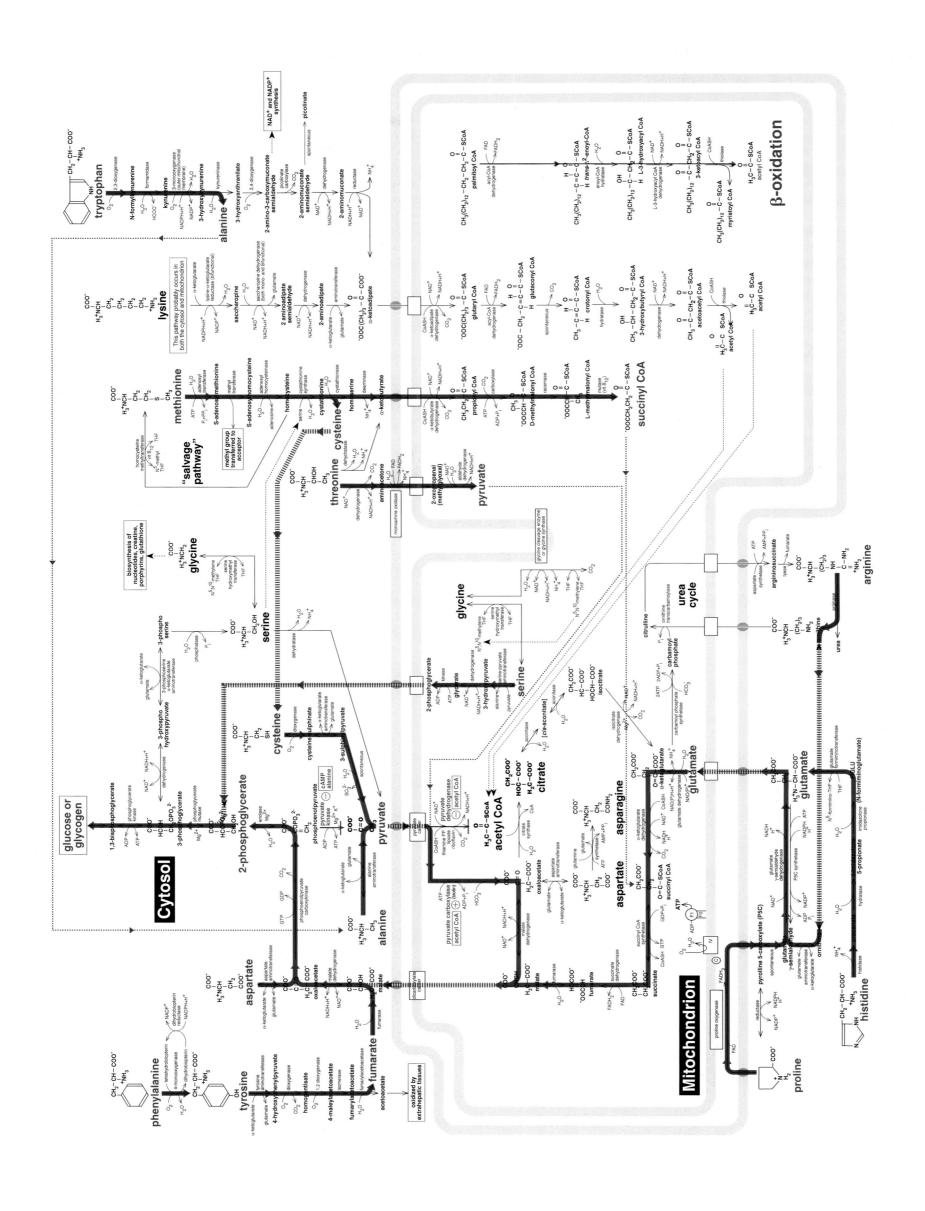

Metabolism of protein to fat

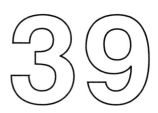

In spite of the exhortation by some popular weight-reducing diets to eat large quantities of protein, it should be remembered that surplus dietary protein can be converted to fat. For protein to be converted to fatty acids and triacylglycerols, the essential precursors for fatty acid synthesis, namely a carbon source, acetyl CoA, and biosynthetic reducing power as NADPH, must be formed.

Chart 39.1 (opposite)
Metabolism of amino acids to triacylglycerol.

Chart 39.1: Metabolism of amino acids to triacylglycerol
Metabolism of protein to acetyl CoA

Dietary protein is digested by gastric and intestinal proteolytic enzymes to form amino acids, which are absorbed into the blood and transported to the liver. Here (with the notable exception of the branched-chain amino acids), transamination with α-ketoglutarate produces glutamate and the corresponding α-ketoacids. The amino nitrogen is detoxified in the form of urea.

The carbon skeletons derived from phenylalanine, tyrosine, threonine, glycine, serine, cysteine, alanine, tryptophan, methionine, valine, isoleucine, glutamate, proline, histidine, aspartate, asparagine and arginine enter the pathways for metabolism to pyruvate as shown in the chart. The pyruvate thus formed enters the mitochondrion and can proceed either via **pyruvate carboxylase** to oxaloacetate, entering the pyruvate/malate cycle (see Chapter 13), or it can be decarboxylated to acetyl CoA by **pyruvate dehydrogenase**.

The ketogenic amino acids (and fragments of the dual, glucogenic/ketogenic amino acids), namely lysine, tryptophan, leucine and isoleucine, are metabolized to acetyl CoA. **NB:** Although phenylalanine and tyrosine, when degraded, yield acetoacetate, this cannot be metabolized by the liver and so is likely to be exported for use as a respiratory fuel elsewhere (see Chapter 28). Since fatty acid synthesis occurs in the cytosol, acetyl CoA is transported from the mitochondrion to the cytosol by a process known as the **pyruvate/malate cycle** (see Chapter 13). This involves the transport of citrate to the cytosol, where it is cleaved by citrate lyase to form oxaloacetate and **acetyl CoA**. The **acetyl CoA** is now available for fatty acid synthesis.

Sources of NADPH
Pyruvate/malate cycle

In Chapter 38, the metabolism of amino acids to glucose in the starved state was described. Furthermore, it was explained that, following refeeding, there is a transitional period during which the liver remains in gluconeogenic mode, notwithstanding the fact that it now has an abundant supply of glucose for glycolysis. Moreover, lipolysis and β-oxidation of fatty acids continue during this transition period. However, in due course following refeeding, insulin, which is secreted by the pancreas, gains hormonal dominance, β-oxidation ceases, and fatty acid synthesis prevails.

Insulin acts by activating pyruvate dehydrogenase, thus promoting the oxidative decarboxylation of pyruvate to acetyl CoA and providing a carbon source for lipogenesis. Insulin also inhibits transcription of the phosphoenolpyruvate carboxykinase (PEPCK) gene. This leads to decreased PEPCK activity, and malate formed from the amino acid precursors can no longer be metabolized via oxaloacetate to phosphoenolpyruvate. Consequently, gluconeogenesis is inhibited. Malate now follows an alternative route and is oxidatively decarboxylated by the **malic enzyme** to form pyruvate and **NADPH**. The pyruvate/malate cycle is described more fully in Chapter 13.

Pentose phosphate pathway

Providing a source of glucose 6-phosphate is available, for example, from dietary glucose or fructose, the pentose phosphate pathway can generate NADPH for fatty acid synthesis. This process is described in Chapter 12.

Esterification of fatty acids to triacylglycerols

Glyceraldehyde 3-phosphate formed by the pentose phosphate pathway is in equilibrium with dihydroxyacetone phosphate, which is reduced by glycerol 3-phosphate dehydrogenase to form glycerol 3-phosphate. This can be used to esterify fatty acids, as described in Chapter 25.

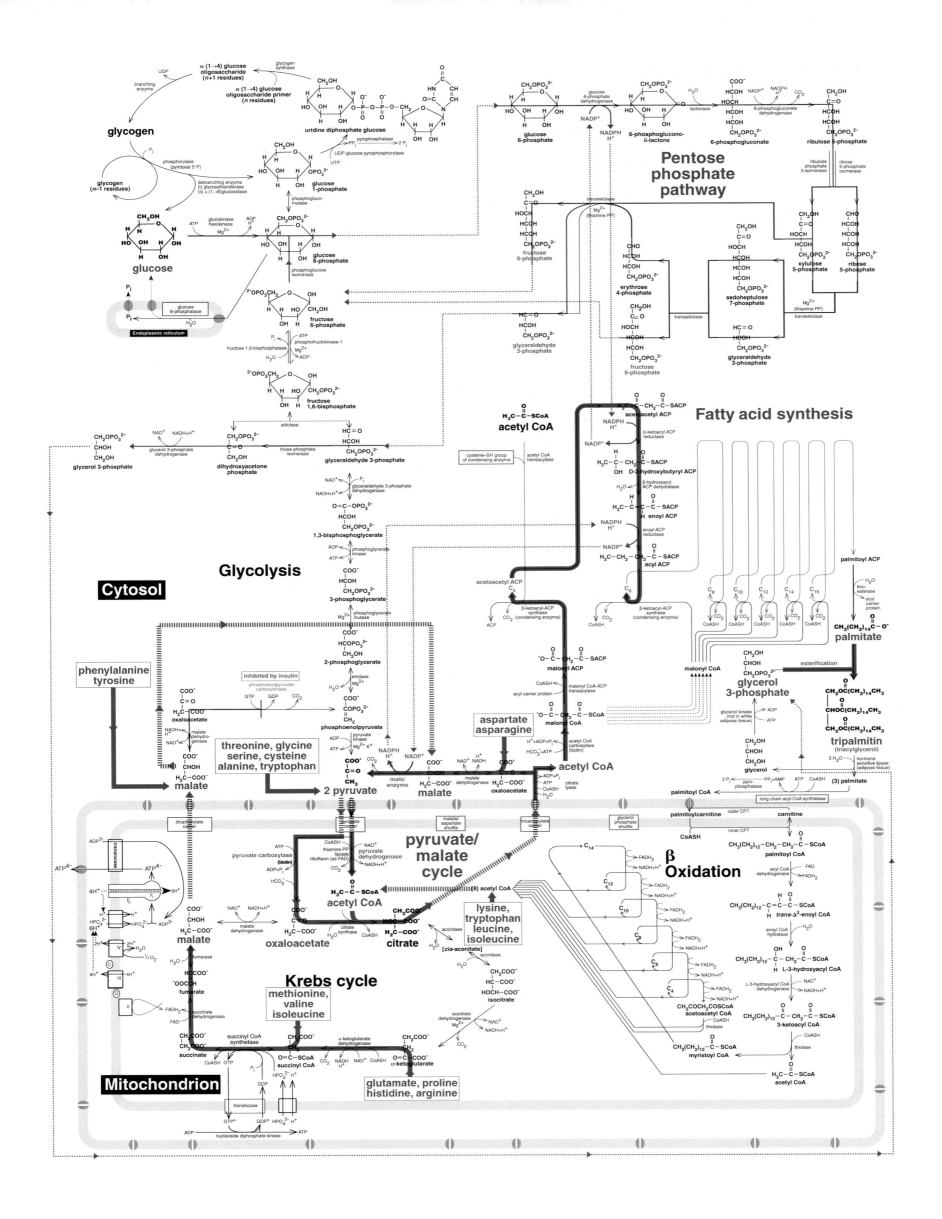

Disorders of amino acid metabolism

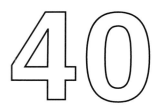

There is a very large body of literature on these rare inborn errors of amino acid metabolism, which has often contributed to our understanding of normal metabolic processes. A few examples are listed below and/or are indicated on the charts.

Phenylketonuria

This is an autosomal recessive disorder resulting from deficiency of **phenylalanine monooxygenase** (also known as phenylalanine hydroxylase) activity. Whereas the monooxygenase is usually directly involved, in 3% of cases the disorder is due to impaired synthesis of its coenzyme, **tetrahydrobiopterin**. Because phenylalanine cannot be metabolized to tyrosine, it accumulates and is transaminated to the 'phenylketone', phenylpyruvate. Phenylketonuria is described in Chapter 41.

Chart 40.1 (opposite) Disorders of amino acid metabolism.

Albinism

Tyrosine is metabolized by tyrosinase in melanocytes to form the pigment, melanin. Deficiency of **tyrosinase** results in albinism.

Alkaptonuria

This autosomal recessive condition is due to deficiency of **homogentisate 1,2-dioxygenase**. Homogentisate accumulates and is excreted in the urine where, under alkaline conditions, it can undergo oxidation and polymerization to form the black pigment, alkapton.

Type I tyrosinaemia

Type I tyrosinaemia is an autosomal recessive disease due to a deficiency of **fumarylacetoacetase**. This causes accumulation of toxic intermediates, in particular fumarylacetoacetate, which causes DNA alkylation and tumour formation, and succinylacetone, which is an inhibitor of porphobilinogen synthase (see Chapter 45). Type I tyrosinaemia is described in Chapter 41.

Treatment of type I tyrosinaemia has been revolutionized using NTBC – 2-(2-nitro-4-trifluoro-methylbenzoyl)-1,3-cyclohexanedione – to inhibit 4-hydroxy-phenylpyruvate dioxygenase. Also, restriction of dietary phenylalanine and tyrosine is necessary.

Non-ketotic hyperglycinaemia

This condition is due to deficiency of **glycine cleavage enzyme** and causes accumulation of glycine in body fluids including the nervous system, where it causes neurological symptoms. This is because glycine can function as a neurotransmitter and potentiates the *N*-methyl-D-aspartate (NMDA) receptor. Consequently, when glycine accumulates, neonates suffer feeding difficulties, myoclonic seizures, hypotonia, and attacks of apnoea. In severe cases they may die or suffer severe neurological disease. In milder forms, patients survive with mental retardation without suffering the other features of the early onset form of the disease. Glycine is an inhibitory neurotransmitter in spinal cords.

Finally, hyperglycinaemia can also occur during valproate therapy.

Histidinaemia

This is an autosomal recessive disorder in which deficiency of **histidase** causes an accumulation of histidine.

Maple syrup urine disease

In this autosomal recessive disorder, deficiency of the **branched-chain α-ketoacid dehydrogenase** complex causes accumulation of the branched-chain amino acids isoleucine, valine and leucine, and their corresponding α-ketoacids, α-methylbutyrate, isobutyrate and isovalerate. These compounds smell like maple syrup, hence the name of this condition. However, some clinicians liken the odour to fenugreek.

Methylmalonic aciduria

This condition is caused by deficiency of L-methylmalonyl CoA reductase or by vitamin B_{12} deficiency, Charts 40.1 and 40.2. Patients suffer lethargy, delayed psychomotor development, seizures and acute encephalopathy. Most die in infancy or childhood.

ß-Hydroxy-ß-methylglutaric aciduria

ß-Hydroxy-ß-methylglutaryl CoA lyase deficiency is an autosomal recessive disorder of leucine catabolism and ketogenesis which is associated with hypoketotic hypoglycaemia, hyperammonaemia and metabolic acidosis.

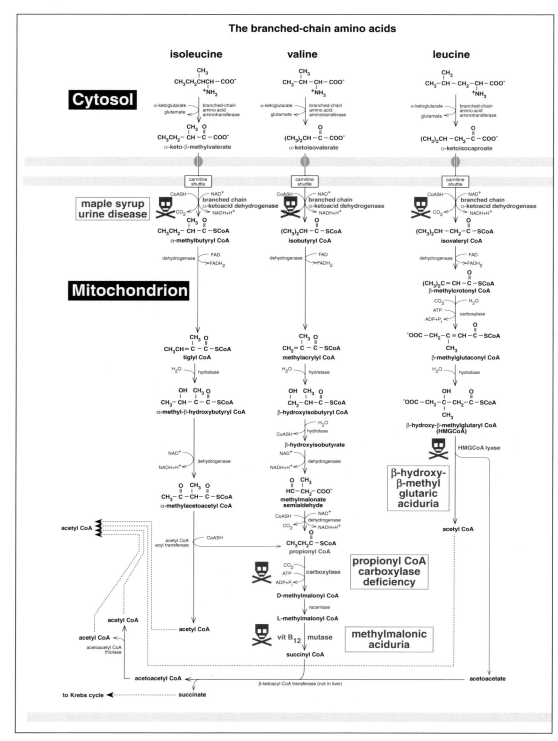

Chart 40.2 Disorders of branched amino acid metabolism.

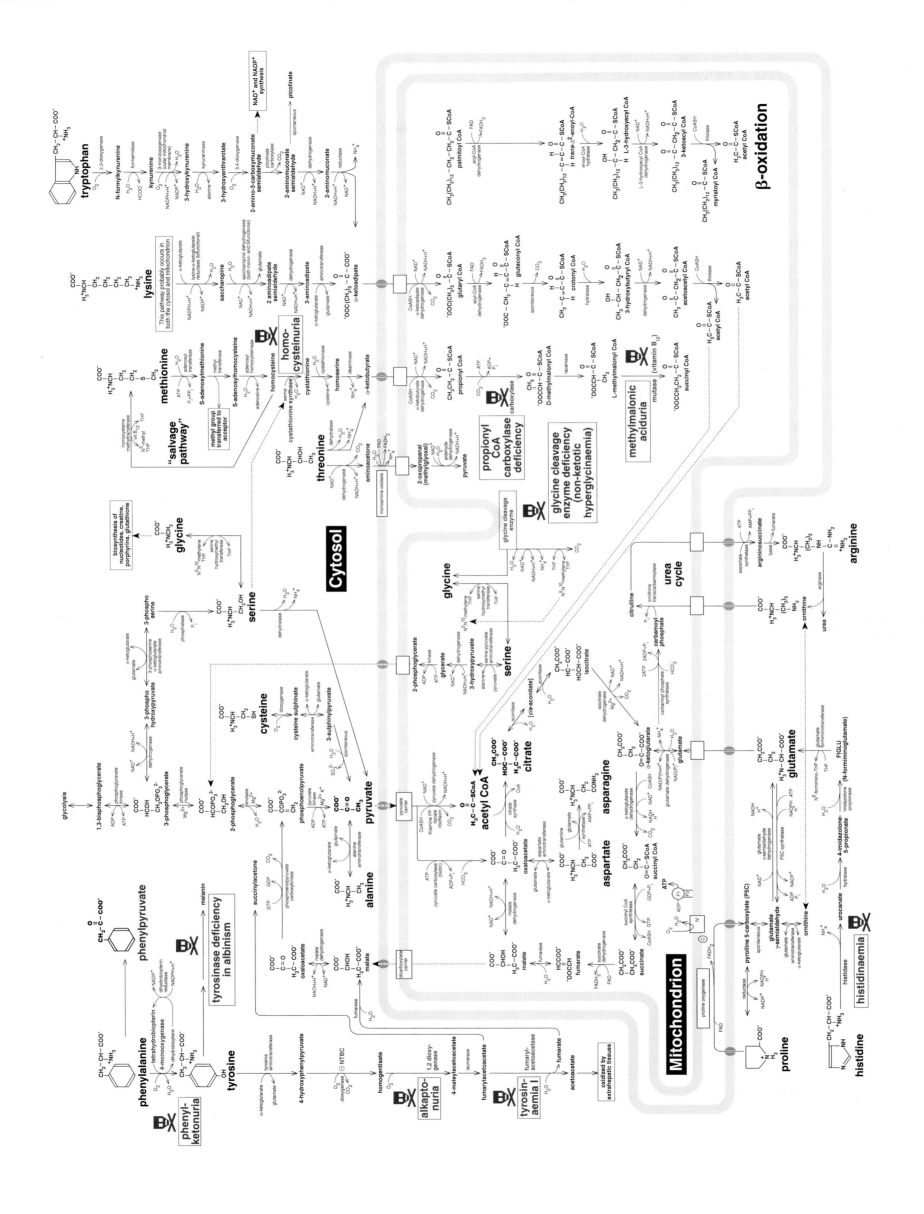

Phenylalanine and tyrosine metabolism

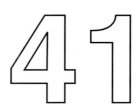

Chart 41.1 (opposite) Phenylalanine and tyrosine metabolism.

Phenylalanine can be hydroxylated to tyrosine, which is the precursor of the pigment melanin; the thyroid hormones thyroxine (T_4) and tri-iodothyronine (T_3); and the catecholamines: dopamine, noradrenaline (norepinephrine) and adrenaline (epinephrine). Any additional phenylalanine or tyrosine surplus to requirement for protein synthesis will be oxidized to acetoacetate and fumarate.

Inborn errors of phenylalanine metabolism

Phenylketonuria (PKU)

This autosomal recessive disorder, the most common inborn error of amino acid metabolism in the UK, is caused by deficiency of **phenylalanine monooxygenase** (also known as **phenylalanine hydroxylase, PAH**). Usually the monooxygenase is directly involved but in 3% of cases the disorder is due to impaired synthesis of its coenzyme, **tetrahydrobiopterin**. In both cases, because tryptophan cannot be metabolized to tyrosine, it accumulates and is transaminated to the phenylketone, **phenylpyruvate**.

PKU patients suffer neurological symptoms and have a low IQ. There are two hypotheses to explain this:

1 **The toxic metabolite hypothesis.** Phenylpyruvate and its metabolite phenyllactate can inhibit metabolic processes. However, they do so only at concentrations greater than those found in PKU patients.

2 **The transport hypothesis.** This proposes that high concentrations of phenylalanine competitively interfere with the transport into the brain of other large neutral amino acids including tryptophan (a precursor of serotonin, see Chapter 42), and tyrosine (a precursor of dopamine, see Chart 41.1 opposite).

Inborn errors of tyrosine metabolism

Tyrosinaemia I (hepatorenal tyrosinaemia)

This is an autosomal recessive disorder of **fumarylacetoacetase**. Patients suffer severe liver disease and develop carcinoma caused by accumulation of the toxic, electrophilic metabolites, **fumarylacetoacetate** and **succinylacetone**, see Chart 41.1 opposite. Succinylacetone can also cause porphyria-like attacks because it is a competitive inhibitor of PBG synthase (Chapter 45). Because oxidation of tyrosine is inhibited, tyrosine is diverted towards the catecholamines which are produced in increased amounts and may cause hypertension. Patients also develop **hypermethioninaemia** and have a 'cabbage-like' odour.

Traditionally, Type I tyrosinaemia was treated with low-tyrosine and low-tryptophan diets and liver transplantation. However, since 1991 a trial of the **4-hydoxyphenylpyruvate oxidase** inhibitor, **NTBC** (2-(2-nitro-4-trifluoromethylbenzoyl)-1,3-cyclohexanedione) plus dietary restriction of tryptophan and tyrosine has been conducted with great success.

NTBC is a weedkiller that, during toxicity trials (for its herbicidal use), caused hypertyrosinaemia in experimental animals. It was shown to inhibit **4-hydroxyphenylpyruvate oxidase.** Then, following inspired and bold lateral thinking (and no doubt much trepidation at the thought of using a weedkiller as a therapeutic drug), it was given to children with tyrosinaemia I, with remarkable results. NTBC stopped the production of fumaryl-acetoacetate and succinylacetone thereby preventing the severe liver damage caused by these hepatotoxins. This clinical trial was successful and in 2002 the FDA approved the use of NTBC.

Tyrosinaemia II (Richner–Hanhart syndrome; oculocutaneous tyrosinaemia)

This is an autosomal recessive disorder of **tyrosine aminotransferase** that affects the eyes, skin and central nervous system. The eye problems are due to accumulation of tyrosine in the cornea. Once diagnosed, this condition is successfully treated and the lesions are reversed with low dietary tyrosine and phenylalanine formulations.

Tyrosinaemia III

This is a very rare autosomal recessive disorder caused by deficiency of **4-hydroxyphenylpyruvate oxidase**. Tyrosine and phenolic metabolites accumulate and patients suffer neurological symptoms and mental retardation.

Hawkinsinuria

This is a rare autosomal dominant disorder caused by a partial defect **of 4-hydroxyphenylpyruvate oxidase** activity. This partial defect prevents the **epoxide** intermediates produced during the reaction (see Chart 41.1) from rearranging to form homogentisate and instead they react with **glutathione** to form **hawkinsin** (which is an amino acid named after the Hawkins family in which the disorder was discovered). Infants present with metabolic acidosis, a body odour 'like a swimming pool', and excrete hawkinsin. They also excrete 5-oxoproline (pyroglutamic acid), presumably secondary to glutathione depletion (see Chapter 12). In later life, they excrete 4-hydroxycyclohexylacetic acid (**HCAA**).

Other inborn errors of tyrosine metabolism

Albinism and alkaptonuria are described in Chapter 40.

Parkinson's disease

This disease, which usually develops from age 60 onwards, is caused by destruction of the brain region, known as the substantia nigra, that produces the neurotransmitter **dopamine**. The symptoms of Parkinson's disease include tremor, muscular rigidity and akinesia. The use of the dopamine precursor **L-DOPA** (levodopa) was a landmark in the treatment of Parkinson's disease, and was subsequently refined by combining it with a peripheral (i.e. extracerebral) **L-DOPA decarboxylase** inhibitor (e.g. carbidopa or benserazide). Other therapeutic drugs used are dopamine agonists and the catechol-*O*-methyltransferase (**COMT**) inhibitors entacapone and tolcapone, which prevent the catabolism of L-DOPA to form **3-OMD** (3-*O*-methyldopa).

Phaeochromocytoma

This rare condition is usually caused by a tumour of the adrenal medulla, which produces excessive amounts of the catecholamines **adrenaline** (epinephrine) and **noradrenaline** (norepinephrine), and their catabolic products **metadrenaline** (metepinephrine), **normetadrenaline** (normetepinephrine) and **VMA** (vanillylmandelic acid) (also known as HMMA (hydroxymethoxmandelic acid)). However, 10% of cases occur in the sympathetic nerve chain and overproduce noradrenaline. If the tumour releases a surge of catecholamines, patients suffer a hypertensive attack associated with severe headache, sweating, palpitations, anxiety, glucosuria and, if adrenaline predominates, tachycardia. The tumour can be surgically removed but handling of the tumour during the operation can cause a surge of catecholamines precipitating a hypertensive crisis. Patients are therefore prepared preoperatively with adrenergic blockers. There are reports that treatment with α-methyl-*p*-tyrosine, which inhibits tyrosine 3-monooxygenase, has been used to deplete the tumour of catecholamines prior to the operation.

Neuroblastoma

This rare tumour usually presents in children less than 5 years old and 70% have metastatic disease at diagnosis. During the last decade, mass screening trials of children were conducted, the outcome of which remains controversial. Urine was dried onto filter paper and used for assays of **HVA** (**homovanillic acid**) and **VMA**, which are excreted in increased amounts in neuroblastoma.

Dopamine and mental illness

The 'dopamine hypothesis' for schizophrenia postulates increased brain dopaminergic activity. Although several research approaches suggest an association of psychosis with altered dopaminergic transmission, the evidence is not conclusive. The *COMT* gene is receiving special attention as a candidate risk-factor for schizophrenia.

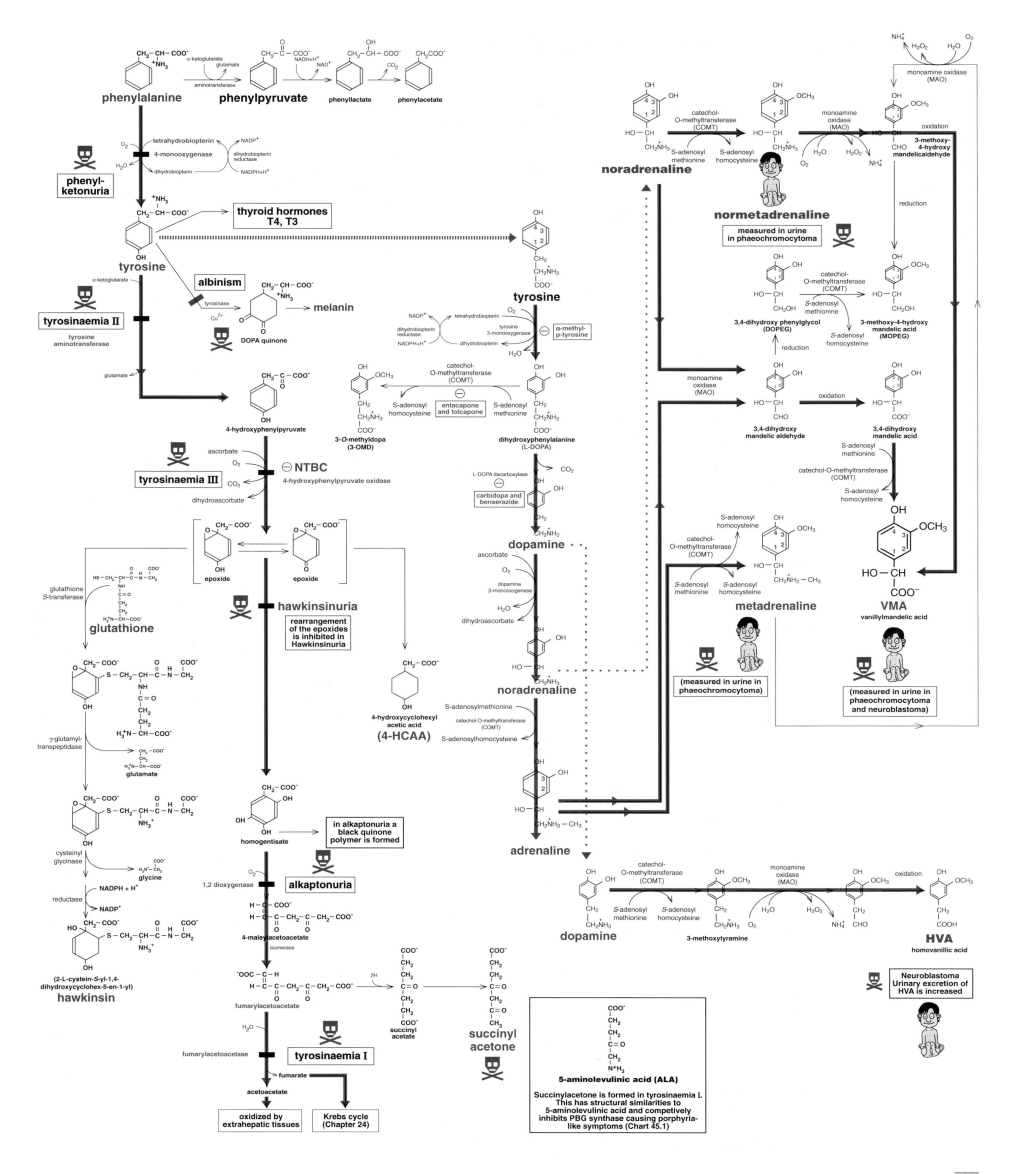

Tryptophan metabolism: the biosynthesis of NAD⁺, serotonin and melatonin

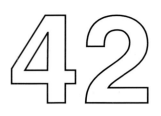

Chart 42.1 (opposite)
Tryptophan metabolism.

Hartnup disease, niacin deficiency and pellagra

Tryptophan is an essential amino acid whose importance is demonstrated in **Hartnup disease**. This is an autosomal recessive disorder in which renal loss and intestinal malabsorption of tryptophan and other neutral amino acids occurs. Patients with Hartnup disease suffer neurological symptoms and skin lesions resembling severe sunburn, which are similar to pellagra. Pellagra is classically seen in dietary **niacin** deficiency, niacin being the collective term for the NAD⁺ precursors **nicotinic acid** and **nicotinamide**. However, tryptophan metabolism via the **kynurenine pathway** also produces precursors of NAD⁺.

The kynurenine pathway

The regulatory enzymes for the kynurenine pathway are **tryptophan 2,3-dioxygenase (TDO)** and the less specific **indoleamine 2,3-dioxygenase (IDO)** (see Chart 42.1).

The production of NAD⁺ and NADP⁺

The kynurenine pathway is the main pathway for tryptophan metabolism and it provides precursors that supplement dietary niacin (i.e. nicotinic acid and nicotinamide) for the biosynthesis of **NAD⁺** and **NADP⁺**. It is generally accepted that 60 mg of tryptophan is equivalent to 1 mg of niacin. Because kynureninase needs **vitamin B_6**, deficiency of the latter can cause secondary pellagra. In a malnourished population with marginally sufficient dietary tryptophan, women of childbearing age are twice as vulnerable as men to suffer pellagra. This is because oestrogens inhibit several enzymes of the kynurenine pathway that produces the precursors of NAD⁺. Conversely, when abundant any tryptophan surplus to requirement is metabolized via α-ketoadipate for ATP production.

Kynurenine and its metabolites prevent maternal rejection of the fetus

Recent studies have suggested that upstream products of the kynurenine pathway may have several important functions, for example, in immunology and regulation of cell proliferation, and the pathway is attracting attention as a target for the development of new drugs. Work in mice suggests that placental trophoblasts produce indoleamine 2,3-dioxygenase (IDO) leading to the production of kynurenine, picolinate and quinolinate, which prevent maternal T cells from activating a lethal anti-fetal response.

The indoleamine pathway for the formation of serotonin (5-hydroxytryptamine) and melatonin

A pathway of major neuroendocrinological importance is the indoleamine pathway, which forms the neurotransmitter **serotonin** and the hormone **melatonin** in the pineal gland and retina (Chart 42.1). Because impaired serotonin metabolism has been associated with the 'affective disorders' (disorders of mood), this pathway has been a target for the treatment of depression. Indeed, tryptophan and 5-hydroxytryptophan have historically been used to treat depression. Also, melatonin has been associated with 'seasonal affective disorder' (SAD) but this remains unproven. This depression is thought to be caused by long winter nights. Many sufferers benefit from light treatment by exposure to 2500 lux for 2 hours each morning.

Depression as a neurochemical disease

Although one in four people experience mental disease each year, it is a sad fact that sufferers are frequently stigmatized, even in the 21st century, because of the debilitating effect it has on their personalities. All too frequently depression is unfairly considered to be self-indulgent weakness due to lack of resolve and determination. This is despite the fact that a psychiatric condition such as **endogenous depression** is a disease with a substantial biochemical component. *Perhaps it is time to refer to these disorders as 'neurochemical' diseases to prevent the stigmatizing effect that 'mental' illness can have on people.*

Of course, not all depression is **primarily** of neurochemical origin. For example, bad news such as failing exams or bereavement will quite naturally cause a period of 'reactive' depression secondary to the tragic event. However, there are people with a contented lifestyle who for no apparent reason slip into a period of inconsolable depression. It is these people who are probably suffering from an 'endogenous' biochemical failure to make sufficient brain serotonin and consequently their brain function is depressed. Clearly, lack of space here permits only a simplistic view of reactive and endogenous depression since it is likely there is an interaction between the two. However, there is an urgent need for an enlightened public attitude to these 'taboo' diseases.

The 'indoleamine-amine hypothesis for affective disease' proposes that brain concentrations of neuroactive amines e.g. serotonin are associated with mood disorders. In depression, there is insufficient serotonin present for neurotransmission so brain function is depressed. Successful treatment of depression with serotonin reuptake inhibitors such as Prozac, which increase synaptic concentrations of serotonin, supports this hypothesis. Conversely, it is hypothesized that excessive concentrations of serotonin cause mania.

Serotonin metabolism

The regulatory enzyme for serotonin biosynthesis is **tryptophan hydroxylase**. Note that tryptophan hydroxylase has to compete for tryptophan with its rivals TDO and IDO. It is possible that if the hydroxylase is insufficiently active, brain concentrations of serotonin can be depleted and this could cause depression.

Catabolism occurs when serotonin is deaminated by monoamine oxidase and then oxidized to **5-hydroxyindoleacetic acid (5-HIAA)**. 5-HIAA is excreted in excessive amounts in patients with carcinoid syndrome.

Melatonin metabolism

Melatonin is made in the pineal gland normally during periods of darkness and is almost undetectable in daylight. The regulatory enzyme is **arylalkylamine N-acetyltransferase (AANAT)**. AANAT is **up-regulated** by noradrenergic stimulation which normally occurs during the **dark phase** of the day. It is **down-regulated by light** which stimulates photoreceptors in the retina and initiates signals that are transmitted through a neural circuit including the **suprachiasmatic nuclei (SCN,** also called the '**biological clock**') and then onwards towards the pineal gland. N.B. During continuous darkness melatonin varies up-and-down driven by the SCN i.e. a light/dark cycle is not needed to produce a rhythm.

Melatonin biosynthesis: AANAT is up-regulated by noradrenaline

Noradrenergic stimulation of primarily β- but also α-adrenergic receptors on pinealocytes activates **protein kinase A (PKA)** which phosphorylates and activates AANAT, Chart 42.1. Phosphorylated AANAT is now protected from degradation by its 'bodyguard' **14-3-3 protein** (named after the laboratory number of the fraction from which it was isolated by its discoverers).

Melatonin biosynthesis: AANAT is down-regulated by light

Light, via the SCN adjusts the time duration of sympathetic input to the pineal which inhibits synthesis of melatonin in the pineal gland. Light causes a rapid decrease in both the activity of AANAT and the amount of AANAT protein, which has a $t_{1/2}$ of 3 minutes. When noradrenergic stimulation ceases, PKA activity also decreases, protein phosphatase dephosphorylates AANAT which loses its protective 14-3-3 protein and is exposed to and destroyed by **proteosomal proteolysis**.

Catabolism of melatonin

Melatonin is hydrophobic and must be conjugated with hydrophilic groups before it can be excreted in the urine. It is metabolized by **CYP 1A2** to **6-hydroxymelatonin** which can be conjugated in two ways. The principal excretory product is **6-sulphatoxymelatonin** with the sulphate donated by **3'-phosphoadenosine-5'-phosphosulphate (PAPS)**. The alternative is conjugation with UDP glucuronate to form **6-hydroxymelatonin glucuronide**.

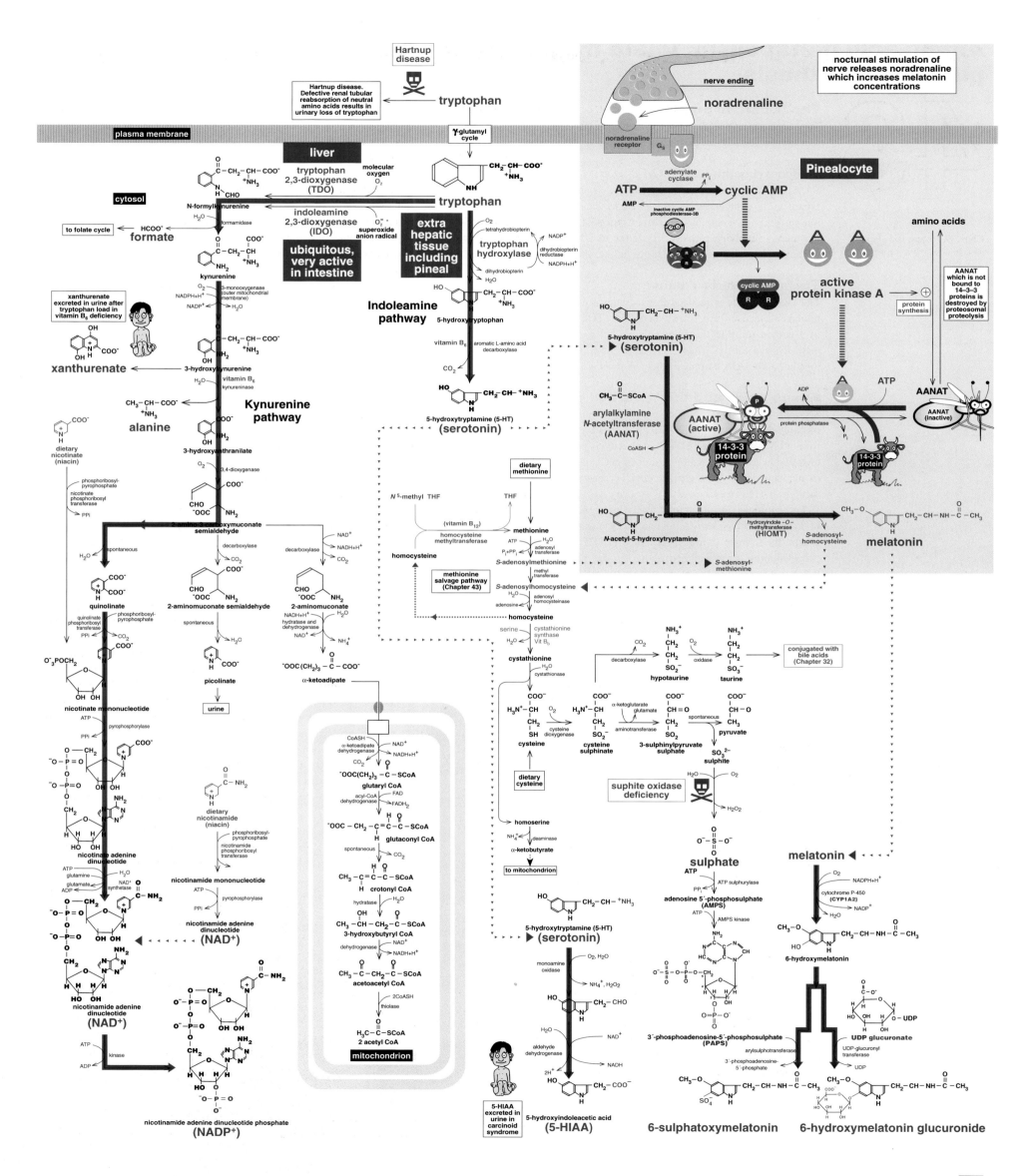

Amino acid metabolism, folate metabolism and the '1-carbon pool' I: purine biosynthesis

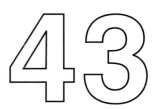

Chart 43.1 (opposite) Purine biosynthesis.

The '1-carbon pool'

This term describes the 1-carbon residues associated with *S*-adenosylmethionine (SAM) and folate that are available for metabolic reactions.

S-adenosylmethionine (SAM)

SAM, which is formed from methionine, is the major donor of methyl groups for biosynthetic reactions. It can, for example, methylate noradrenaline to form adrenaline, as shown in Chart 43.1 opposite. Other important reactions involving SAM include the methylation of phosphatidylethanolamine to phosphatidylcholine, and the formation of creatine.

The folate '1-carbon' units

The vitamin folate is reduced in two stages by dihydrofolate reductase to produce the active form, **tetrahydrofolate** (THF). THF is a versatile carrier of 1-carbon units in the following oxidation states: methyl, methylene, methenyl and formyl. These THF compounds, which are interconvertible, together with SAM, comprise what is known as the '1-carbon pool'.

Amino acids and the '1-carbon pool'

Serine is converted to **glycine**, in a reaction catalysed by **serine hydroxymethyl transferase**, with the transfer of a methyl group to the THF so as to form N^5,N^{10}-**methylene THF**. This reaction is particularly important in the thymidylate synthase reaction described in Chapter 44. Oxidation of glycine in mitochondria by the glycine cleavage enzyme also produces N^5,N^{10}-methylene THF (see Chapter 37).

   Tryptophan is oxidized to *N*-formylkynurenine, which, in the presence of formamidase, yields kynurenine and the toxic product **formate**. THF accepts the formate, producing N^{10}-**formyl THF**.

   Methionine, as mentioned above, is the precursor of SAM, which, following transfer of the methyl group, forms homocysteine. Methionine can be regenerated from homocysteine by methylation using N^5-methyl THF in a salvage pathway. **NB:** This reaction, catalysed by homocysteine methyltransferase, requires **vitamin B$_{12}$**, and lack of this vitamin can lead to folate being caught in the 'methyl–folate' trap (see below).

Amino acid metabolism and purine synthesis

Glycine contributes the C-4, C-5 and N-7 atoms to the purine ring in a reaction catalysed by glycinamide ribonucleotide (GAR) synthetase (see Chart 43.1 opposite).

   Aspartate is an important donor of nitrogen atoms during purine biosynthesis, contributing the N-1 atom to the purine ring, and the –NH$_2$ group in the adenylosuccinate synthetase reaction of the pathway that forms AMP from inosine monophosphate (IMP) (see Chart 43.2 below).

Glutamine plays a very important role in nucleotide metabolism. It donates the nitrogen atoms that form N-9 and N-3 of the purine ring. It also participates in the amination of xanthine monophosphate (XMP) to form guanosine monophosphate (GMP) (see Chart 43.2).

Biosynthesis of purines

Purine nucleotides can be synthesized *de novo*. They can also be reclaimed from existing nucleosides by the so-called 'salvage pathway' (see Chapter 44). The *de novo* pathway needs '1-carbon' units from the folate pool, and several amino acids as detailed below.

De novo pathway for purine biosynthesis

The pathway starts with **ribose 5-phosphate** formed by the pentose phosphate pathway (see Chart 43.1). This is activated to form **phosphoribosyl pyrophosphate** (**PRPP**). A total of 11 reactions are needed to form **IMP** (inosine monophosphate or inosinic acid), which is the precursor of the adenine- and guanine-containing nucleotides. The important roles of glutamine and aspartate as amino donors are emphasized. A total of **three glutamine** molecules and **one aspartate** molecule are needed for the synthesis of GMP. Similarly, a total of **two glutamine** and **two aspartate** molecules are needed for AMP synthesis. A molecule of **glycine** is needed in each case.

   The *de novo* pathway is controlled by feedback inhibition of PRPP amidotransferase by AMP and GMP. In **primary gout** this feedback control is impaired, causing increased production of purines resulting in the increased formation of their sparingly soluble excretory product, uric acid.

Vitamin B$_{12}$ and the 'methyl-folate trap'

Vitamin B$_{12}$, or more precisely its methyl cobalamin derivative, is an essential coenzyme for the transfer of methyl groups in the **methionine salvage pathway** (see Chart 43.1). Accordingly, in B$_{12}$ deficiency, THF cannot be released and remains trapped as N^5-methyl THF. Eventually, all the body's folate becomes trapped in the N^5-methyl THF form, and so folate deficiency develops secondary to B$_{12}$ deficiency. Because blood cells turn over rapidly, they need nucleotides for nucleic acid synthesis and are vulnerable to folate deficiency, which causes megaloblastic anaemia. Another effect of folate/B$_{12}$ deficiency is increased plasma concentration of homocysteine, which is associated with cardiovascular disease.

   The methyl-folate trap hypothesis explains the observation that, although the haematological symptoms of B$_{12}$ deficiency respond to folate treatment, the neurological degeneration progresses. Remember that the other enzyme for which B$_{12}$ is a coenzyme is methylmalonyl CoA mutase (see Chapters 36 & 37). Accumulation of methylmalonyl CoA may interfere with the biosynthesis of lipids needed for the myelin sheath.

Chart 43.2
Conversion of IMP to ATP. IMP reacts with aspartate in the presence of GTP to form adenylosuccinate, which is cleaved to form fumarate and AMP. The AMP can be phosphorylated to ADP, which undergoes oxidative phosphorylation to form ATP.

Conversion of IMP to GTP. IMP is oxidized to xanthine monophosphate (XMP), which is aminated to form GMP, which is phosphorylated to form GDP. GDP is phosphorylated by ATP in a reaction catalysed by nucleoside diphosphate kinase. Alternatively, when Krebs cycle is active, GTP is formed from GDP by succinyl CoA synthetase.

Formation of dATP (deoxyadenosine triphosphate) and dGTP (deoxyguanosine triphosphate). The deoxyribonucleotides dATP and dGTP are formed by first reducing ADP and GDP to dADP and dGDP in the presence of ribonucleotide reductase. These are subsequently phosphorylated to form dATP and dGTP, which can be used for the synthesis of DNA.

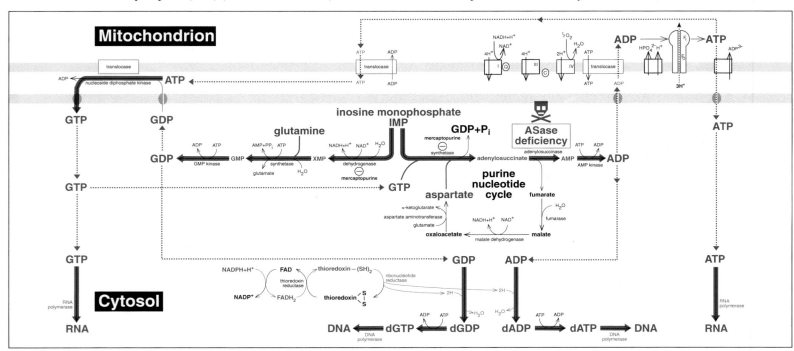

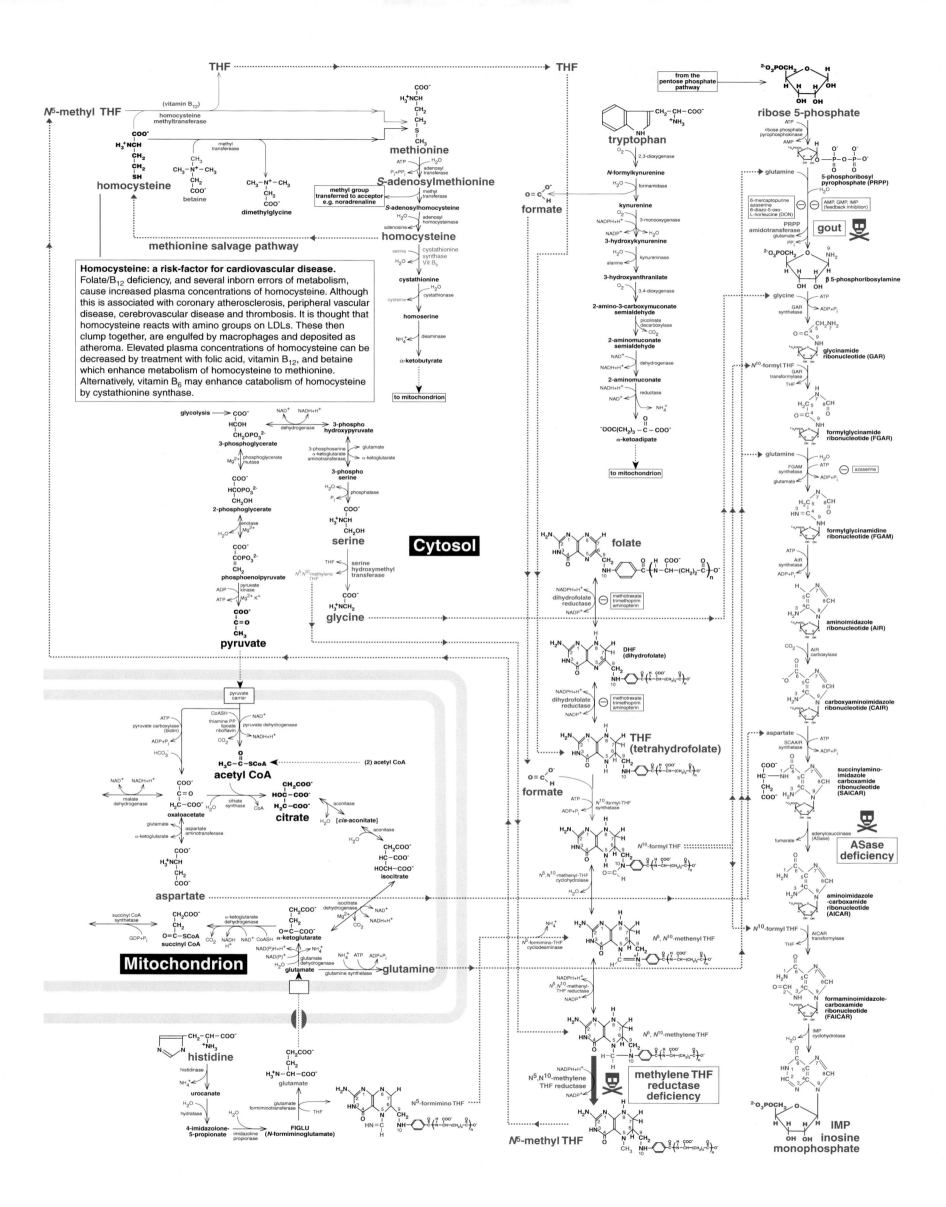

Amino acid metabolism, folate metabolism and the '1-carbon pool' II: pyrimidine biosynthesis

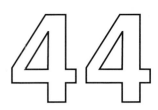

Chart 44.1 (opposite)
Biosynthesis of pyrimidines.

Amino acid metabolism and pyrimidine biosynthesis

The pyrimidine ring is derived from glutamine, aspartate and bicarbonate. The first reaction, catalysed by **carbamoyl phosphate synthetase II (CPS II)**, occurs in the cytosol and produces **carbamoyl phosphate** from bicarbonate, glutamine and two molecules of ATP. This is similar to the mitochondrial reaction involved in the urea cycle, which differs in that it forms carbamoyl phosphate from bicarbonate and NH_4^+ ions. Another difference is that CPS II does not require N-acetyl glutamate as an allosteric stimulator. The rest of the pyrimidine ring is donated by aspartate and, after ring closure and oxidation, **orotate** is formed. It is at this stage that **phosphoribosyl pyrophosphate (PRPP)** is added to yield **orotidine monophosphate (OMP)**, which, following decarboxylation, produces **uridine monophosphate (UMP)**, which is the common precursor of the pyrimidine-containing nucleotides.

Conversion of UMP to UTP and CTP

UMP is phosphorylated by a specific UMP kinase to form uridine diphosphate (UDP), which in turn is phosphorylated by the non-specific nucleoside diphosphate kinase to yield **uridine triphosphate (UTP)**. When UTP is aminated, **cytidine triphosphate (CTP)** is formed.

Formation of deoxycytidine triphosphate (dCTP) and deoxythymidine triphosphate (dTTP)

dCTP is formed from CDP by ribonucleotide reductase, as described for the production of the purine-containing deoxyribonucleotides in Chapter 43.

The pathway for the formation of dTTP is quite distinct from that used to produce dATP, dGTP and dCTP. The pathway starts with dCDP, which is dephosphorylated and deaminated to yield deoxyuridine monophosphate (dUMP). This is methylated by N^5,N^{10}-methylene THF, which is oxidized to dihydrofolate (DHF) in the reaction catalysed by **thymidylate synthase**, and deoxythymidine monophosphate (dTMP) is formed. The dTMP is now phosphorylated by dTMP kinase and nucleoside diphosphate kinase to produce dTTP.

Let us return to the DHF, which is formed by the **thymidylate synthase** reaction. This is reduced by **dihydrofolate reductase**, which regenerates **tetrahydrofolate (THF)**. The cycle is completed when this THF participates in the **serine hydroxymethyltransferase** reaction, which produces glycine and N^5,N^{10}-methylene THF; the latter is now available once more for the thymidylate synthase reaction.

Cancer chemotherapy

Because rapidly dividing cancer cells have a great demand for DNA synthesis, much attention has been directed at the pathways for nucleotide synthesis as a target for chemotherapeutic intervention. These drugs are classified by pharmacologists as 'antimetabolites' and fall into the following categories: glutamine antagonists, folate antagonists, antipyrimidines and antipurines.

Glutamine antagonists

The importance of glutamine for the biosynthesis of purines and pyrimidines has been emphasized already (see Chapter 43). Azaserine and diazo-oxonorleucine (DON) irreversibly inhibit the enzymes involved in the glutamine-utilizing reactions (see Chart 43.1), and reduce the supply of DNA available to cancer cells.

Folate antagonists

Methotrexate, which is a close structural analogue of folate, inhibits **DHF reductase**. This prevents the reduction of DHF to THF, as shown in the chart opposite. Consequently, in the absence of THF, serine hydroxymethyltransferase is unable to generate the N^5,N^{10}-methylene-THF needed by thymidylate synthase for dTMP production.

The clinical benefit to patients treated with high doses of methotrexate is enhanced by the use of folinic acid, N^5-formyl THF (also known as **leucovorin**), which 'rescues' normal cells from the toxic effects of methotrexate.

Antipyrimidines

Fluorouracil inhibits thymidylate synthase and thus prevents the conversion of dUMP to dTMP.

Antipurines

Mercaptopurine inhibits purine biosynthesis at several stages. It inhibits PRPP-amidotransferase (see Chart 43.1), IMP dehydrogenase and adenylosuccinate synthetase (see Chart 43.2).

Salvage pathways for the recycling of purines and pyrimidines

When nucleic acids and nucleotides are degraded, the free purine and pyrimidine bases are formed. These can be recycled by 'salvage pathways', which require much less ATP compared with the energy-intensive de novo pathways shown in Charts 43.1 and 44.1. The salvage pathways require specific **phosphoribosyl transferases (PRTs)** which transfer **PRPP (5-phosphoribosyl pyrophosphate)** in reactions analogous to that of **orotate PRT** (see chart opposite).

AMP salvage

$$\text{adenine} + \text{PRPP} \xrightarrow{\text{adenine PRT}} \text{AMP} + \text{PP}_i$$

IMP and GMP salvage

Both hypoxanthine and guanine can be used as substrates by the enzyme involved:

$$\text{hypoxanthine} + \text{PRPP} \xrightarrow[\substack{\text{hypoxanthine–}\\\text{guanine PRT}}]{\text{Lesch-Nyhan}} \text{IMP} + \text{PP}_i$$

$$\text{guanine} + \text{PRPP} \longrightarrow \text{GMP} + \text{PP}_i$$

UMP and TMP salvage

$$\text{uracil} + \text{PRPP} \xrightarrow{\quad\quad\quad\quad} \text{UMP} + \text{PP}_i$$

$$\text{thymine} + \text{PRPP} \xrightarrow{\text{uracil–thymine PRT}} \text{TMP} + \text{PP}_i$$

NB: Uracil-thymine PRT cannot use cytosine as a substrate.

Lesch–Nyhan syndrome

This is an extremely rare disorder caused by almost total deficiency of **hypoxanthine-guanine PRT**. In this condition, which is characterized by severe self-mutilation, the salvage pathway is inactive. Consequently, the free purines hypoxanthine and guanine are instead oxidized by xanthine oxidase to uric acid which is sparingly soluble and causes gout.

The antiviral drug AZT (azidothymidine)

AZT is an analogue of thymidine that can be phosphorylated to form the nucleotide triphosphate, azidothymidine triphosphate (AZTTP).

AZTTP inhibits the viral DNA polymerase, which is an RNA-dependent polymerase. The host cell's DNA-dependent polymerase is relatively insensitive to inhibition by AZTTP.

Methotrexate

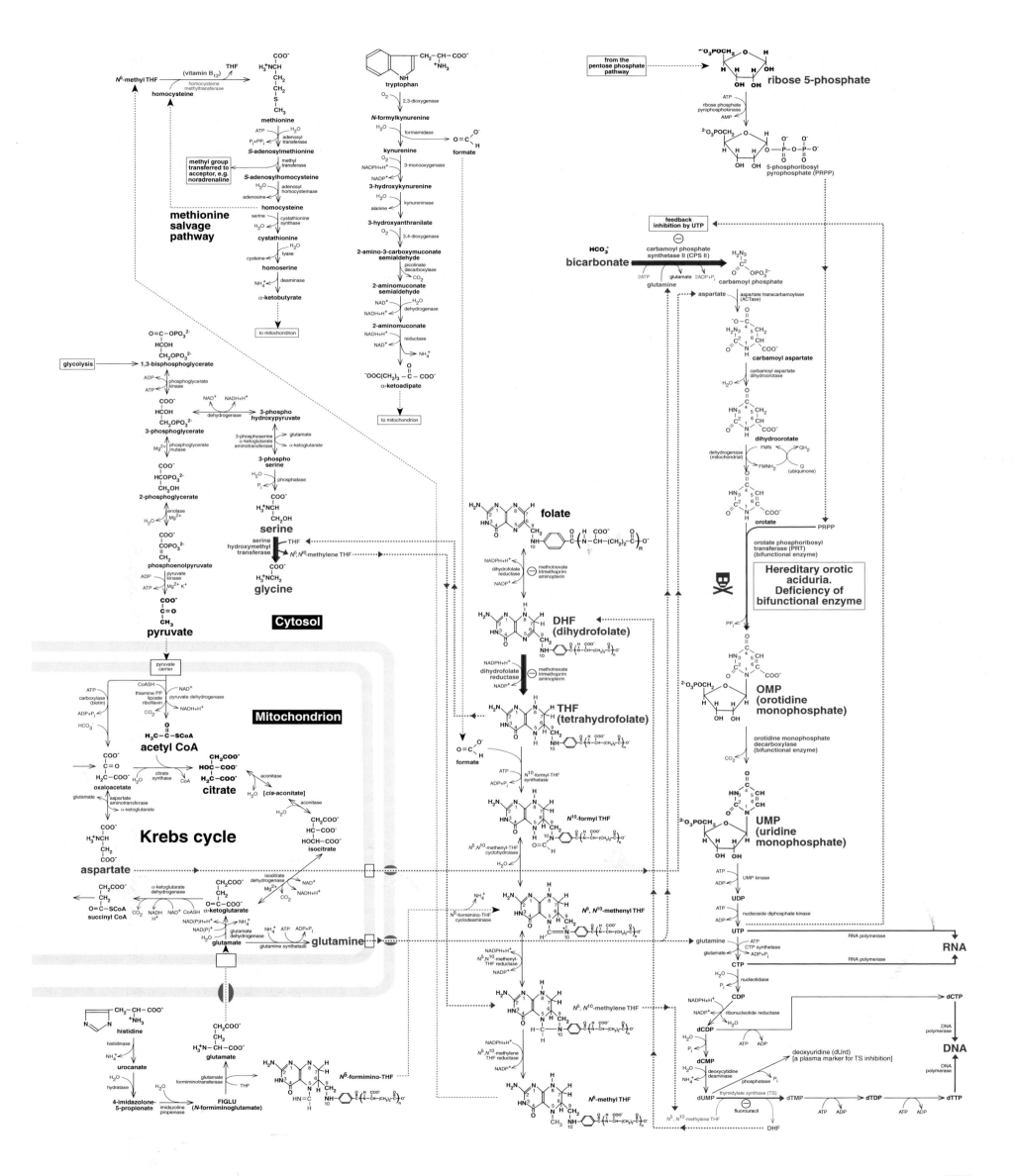

Porphyrin metabolism, haem and the bile pigments

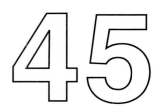

Chart 45.1 (opposite) Biosynthesis of haem and its catabolism to the bile pigments.

Haem biosynthesis

The porphyrin–iron complex, haem, is a component of the cytochromes (e.g. those of the respiratory chain and cytochrome P450, or CYP, family), several enzymes, myoglobin and haemoglobin. Haem is therefore formed in most cells but especially in erythropoietic bone marrow and liver. The latter are particularly affected in the porphyrin disorders, which can be classified as 'erythroid' and 'hepatic' porphyrias respectively.

Succinyl CoA and glycine condense to form **5-aminolevulinic acid (ALA)** in a reaction catalysed by **ALA synthase**, which is the regulatory enzyme for haem biosynthesis. Two molecules of ALA combine to form the monopyrrole, **porphobilinogen (PBG)**. Four molecules of the latter react to form the tetrapyrrole **hydroxymethylbilane**, which cyclizes in a reaction catalysed by uroporphyrinogen III cosynthase to form **uroporphyrinogen III**. Note that hydroxymethylbilane can also cyclize non-enzymically to form an isomer, **uroporphyrinogen I**, differing in the positions of the propionic and acetic acid substituents in the D ring.

Disorders of porphyrin metabolism: 'the porphyrias'

There is a principle common to many of the porphyrias. The porphyrin pathway is regulated by feedback back inhibition of ALA synthase by haem. If an enzyme in this pathway is deficient, the consequent tendency for the haem concentration to fall is compensated by derepression of ALA synthase thus favouring haem biosynthesis. This causes moderately increased concentrations of the metabolites upstream of the enzyme deficiency and maintains haem formation without affecting the subject; i.e. the disorder is 'clinically silent'. A crisis occurs if the patient takes drugs (such as barbiturates, sex steroids or ethanol), which can dramatically increase the activity of ALA synthase. This results in a massive surge of intermediates, which accumulate proximally to the deficient enzyme causing distressing symptoms.

The neurological or photosensitizing effects of metabolites in porphyria

Deficiency of PBG deaminase results in a chronic, but clinically silent, accumulation of PBG and ALA. An acute crisis is precipitated by ingestion of ethanol or drugs, which can cause up to a 50-fold increase in ALA synthase activity. The consequent dramatic increase in these porphyrin precursors is associated with the onset of the **neuropsychiatric** features of the acute crisis, which may be caused by a neurotoxic effect of ALA. Nowadays, it is thought that an acute porphyria was responsible for the bizarre behaviour of King George III towards the end of his reign (1760–1820), which led to the Regency Period following the appointment of his son George as Prince Regent in 1811.

If the enzyme deficiency is after PBG deaminase, then **photosensitivity** is a major feature. This is because porphyrinogens accumulate and are oxidized non-enzymically to their corresponding porphyrins. The latter are activated by light and generate singlet oxygen, which is very cytotoxic and causes the dermatological features of porphyria.

Porphyrin metabolism and the treatment of cancer by photodynamic therapy (PDT)

In the late 1970s Dougherty and coworkers turned to advantage the photosensitizing effects of porphyrins, which cause such distress to patients with porphyria. They pioneered a new form of cancer therapy that exploits this photosensitivity to kill cancer cells by a treatment known as **photodynamic therapy (PDT)**.

Brown and colleagues in England have developed PDT to treat skin tumours by applying 5-aminolevulinic acid topically and then irradiating the site with light of a suitable wavelength. The mechanism is unknown and the following explanation is hypothetical. The final reaction in haem biosynthesis involves **ferrochelatase**, which has a relatively low activity. Accordingly, in the presence of a big load of ALA, protoporphyrin IX accumulates. The latter is a photosensitizer and, when activated by light, produces a photochemical reaction generating singlet oxygen, which results in damage to the cancer cells. Selective targeting of the cancer cells is favoured because, compared with normal tissue, porphobilinogen deaminase activity is relatively high in the cancer cells, whereas ferrochelatase activity is relatively low. These altered activities fortuitously favour accumulation of protoporphyrin IX in the tumour.

Research is in progress to develop lipid-soluble derivatives of levulinic acid with enhanced uptake by the tumour. Another approach is to enhance efficacy by using inhibitors of ferrochelatase such as the specific iron chelator, desferrioxamine.

Catabolism of haem to bilirubin

Following the death, damage or turnover of cells, the various haem proteins (cytochromes, enzymes, haemoglobin and myoglobin) are degraded to release haem from the particular proteins. The cyclic tetrapyrrole ring of haem is split at the α-methene bridge by **haem oxygenase** in a reaction that liberates iron, forms the green linear tetrapyrrole called **biliverdin** and, curiously, emits carbon monoxide. Next, the methene bridge between the C and D rings is reduced to a methane bridge and the major orange/brown bile pigment **bilirubin** is formed. Bilirubin is **hydrophobic** and binds to albumin for transport in the blood to the liver (obviously, this stage is not necessary for bilirubin derived from haem *in situ* in the liver). At the hepatocyte surface bilirubin changes its means of transport for a protein called ligandin, which carries it to the endoplasmic reticulum. Here, it conjugates with two molecules of UDP glucuronide forming bilirubin diglucuronide, which is **hydrophilic**. Bilirubin diglucuronide is secreted in the bile and is further metabolized by the intestinal flora to urobilinogen, urobilin and stercobilin.

Treatment of neonatal jaundice with Sn (tin)-mesoporphyrin

Although mild, transient neonatal jaundice is common and is not usually cause for concern, severe neonatal jaundice caused, for example, by immune haemolysis or glucose 6-phosphate dehydrogenase deficiency (Chapter 12) can be life-threatening, as explained below.

In Chart 45.1 we see how the iron-containing protoporphyrin, haem, is metabolized to bilirubin, which is a **hydrophobic**, fat-soluble molecule. Bilirubin normally combines with UDP-glucuronate to form a **hydrophilic** conjugate prior to excretion in the bile. However, in infants, especially the premature, the conjugating **enzyme UDP-glucuronyl transferase** can be insufficiently developed and so the unconjugated, fat-soluble form of bilirubin accumulates causing neonatal jaundice. In extreme hyperbilirubinaemia, the fat-soluble bilirubin is toxic to the brain causing kernicterus (brain jaundice). Fortunately, hyperbilirubinaemia can often be treated by light therapy, which destroys the bilirubin. However, if this is not successful then exchange transfusion is needed. Recently, there are reports that **Sn-mesoporphyrin** can help avoid the latter.

Sn-mesoporphyrin is a tin-containing metalloporphyrin derived from Sn-protoporphyrin by reducing the vinyl groups at C-2 and C-4 to ethyl groups. It is a potent competitive inhibitor of haem oxygenase thereby restricting formation of bilirubin, and it has been used to treat neonatal jaundice. Of particular note it has been used to treat babies of Jehovah's Witness parents who opposed exchange transfusion on religious grounds.

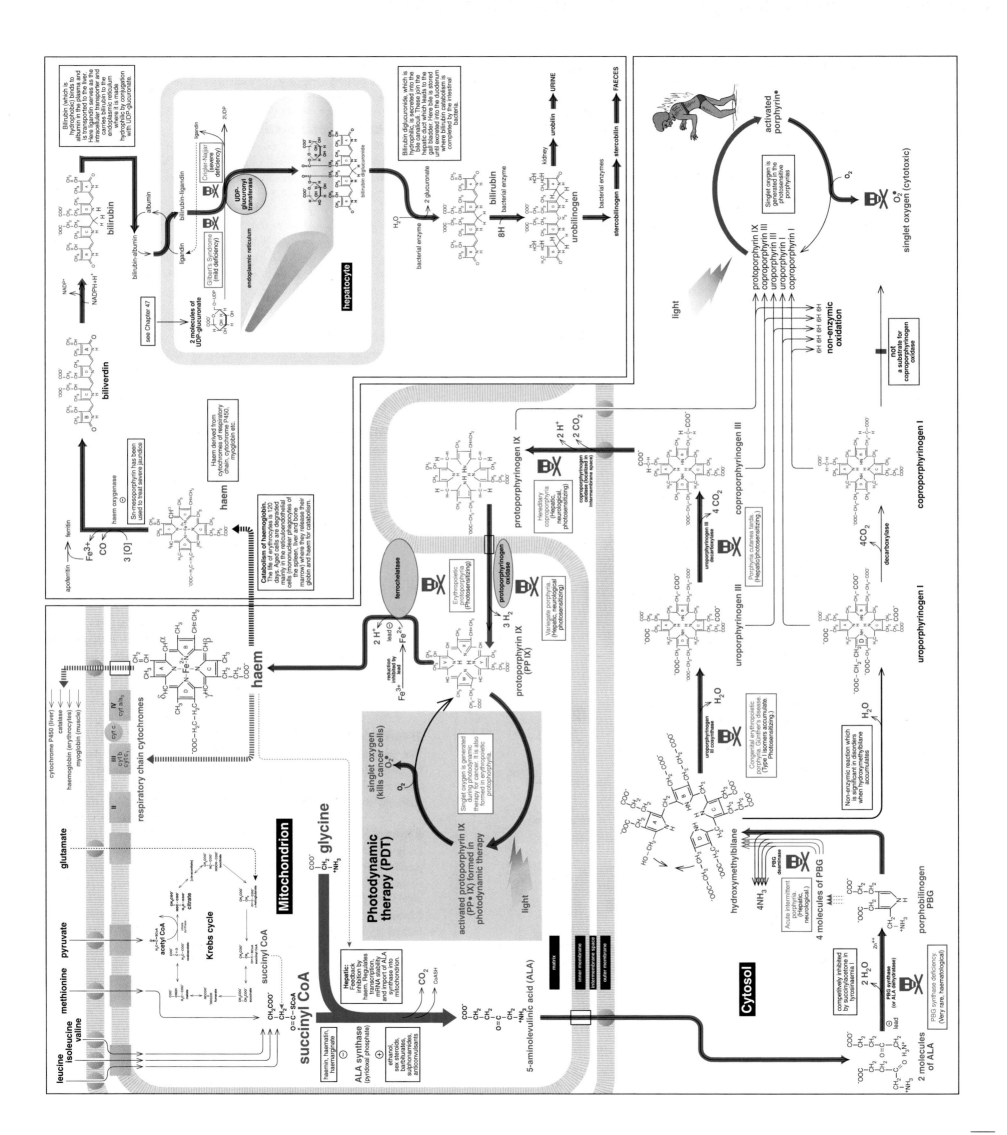

Metabolism of ethanol

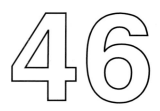

Alcohol, or more precisely ethanol, is a popular mood-altering compound that has been consumed over the centuries as wine, beer and, more recently, as spirits. Whereas there is evidence to suggest that the intake of small quantities of ethanol with food can be beneficial, excessive consumption can cause cirrhosis of the liver, or metabolic disturbances including fatty liver and hypoglycaemia.

Chart 46.1 (opposite)
Metabolism of ethanol.

Ethanol is metabolized by three enzyme systems
Ethanol is rapidly oxidized in the liver by three enzyme systems, but the relative physiological importance of these is not clear (see Diagram 46.1 & Chart 46.1). All three systems produce acetaldehyde, which is normally oxidized rapidly to acetate.

Alcohol dehydrogenase in the cytosol
There may be up to 20 different isoenzymes of alcohol dehydrogenase. The rate of this pathway is largely regulated by the availability of NAD^+. This in turn depends on the ability of the malate/aspartate shuttle (see Chapter 4) to transport reducing equivalents into the mitochondrion and, moreover, on the ability of the respiratory chain to oxidize NADH to NAD^+.

Microsomal ethanol-oxidizing system (MEOS)
Diagram 46.1 The three enzyme systems responsible for ethanol metabolism.

This system is located in the smooth endoplasmic reticulum and involves a cytochrome P450 enzyme. These are a family of monooxygenases concerned with the detoxification of ingested drugs and xenobiotics.

Peroxisomal oxidation of ethanol
Catalase uses hydrogen peroxide to oxidize alcohols such as methanol and ethanol to their corresponding aldehydes.

Metabolism of acetaldehyde
The acetaldehyde formed by any of the three systems mentioned above must now enter the mitochondrion for further oxidation by aldehyde dehydrogenase to form acetate. Finally this acetate could, theoretically, be activated to acetyl CoA for oxidation by Krebs cycle. However, in liver, Krebs cycle is unable to oxidize this acetyl CoA, as we will see below, because of the prevailing high ratio of $NADH/NAD^+$ in the mitochondrial matrix. Consequently the acetate will probably leave the liver for oxidation by the extrahepatic tissues. Evidence suggests that accumulation of acetaldehyde may be responsible for some of the unpleasant effects caused by drinking ethanol, for example, the flushing and nausea that is often seen in those people (45% of Japanese and Chinese) who are genetically deficient in aldehyde dehydrogenase. This phenomenon is used to discourage drinking in alcoholics. They are given disulfiram (Antabuse), which inhibits aldehyde dehydrogenase causing the accumulation of acetaldehyde if ethanol is consumed. Finally, the sulphonylurea drug chlorpropamide inhibits aldehyde dehydrogenase and is known to cause 'chlorpropamide alcohol flushing' in diabetic patients treated with this drug.

The biochemical effects of ethanol
Increased $NADH/NAD^+$ ratio
Following ingestion of ethanol, the cytosolic **alcohol dehydrogenase** reaction and the mitochondrial **aldehyde dehydrogenase** reaction both produce NADH, with relative depletion of NAD^+ so that the ratio of $NADH/NAD^+$ is significantly increased. This has the following effects:
1 **Gluconeogenesis is inhibited.** As shown in the chart opposite, the high $NADH/NAD^+$ ratio in the cytosol displaces the equilibrium of the dehydrogenase reactions in favour of the reduced reactant. In particular, **pyruvate** is reduced to **lactate**, and **oxaloacetate** is reduced to **malate**, thereby preventing the flow of metabolites in the direction of gluconeogenesis. This can cause hypoglycaemia (see below).
2 **Krebs cycle is inhibited in liver.** The high $NADH/NAD^+$ ratio in the mitochondrial matrix prevents the oxidation of **isocitrate** to **α-ketoglutarate**, of α-ketoglutarate to **succinyl CoA**, and of **malate** to **oxaloacetate**. Consequently, although acetate can be activated to acetyl CoA for metabolism in the liver, it is more likely that acetate will be exported for metabolism by the extrahepatic tissues.

Hyperlactataemia and gout
The accumulation of lactate results in hyperlactataemia. This can cause hyperuricaemia because lactate and urate share, and so compete for, the same mechanism for renal tubular secretion. Gout occurs when uric acid, sparingly soluble in plasma, crystallizes in the joints, particularly the toes.

Ethanol interactions with drugs
Long-term treatment with many drugs, for example the barbiturates, causes proliferation of the smooth endoplasmic reticulum and increases the activity of the cytochrome P450 isoenzymes involved in their metabolism and clearance from the body. Similarly, chronic ingestion of excessive quantities of ethanol causes increased proliferation of the endoplasmic reticulum and induction of these enzymes. This means that a sober alcoholic patient will metabolize and inactivate these drugs very rapidly and may need higher than normal doses for treatment. However, in the drunken alcoholic, ethanol preferentially competes with these drugs for metabolism by the cytochrome P450 isoenzymes. As a result, the inactivation and clearance of the barbiturates is suppressed, with the risk of lethal consequences.

Ethanol-induced fasting hypoglycaemia
This condition develops in chronically malnourished individuals several hours after a heavy drinking binge. This is caused by the inhibition of gluconeogenesis, as described above.

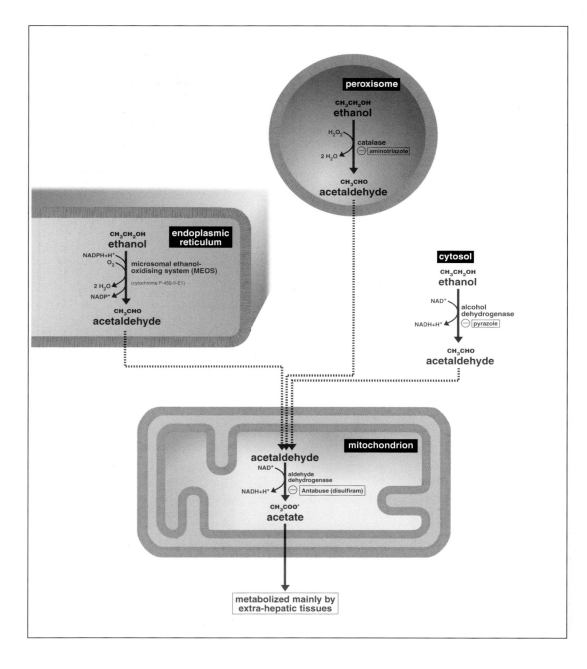

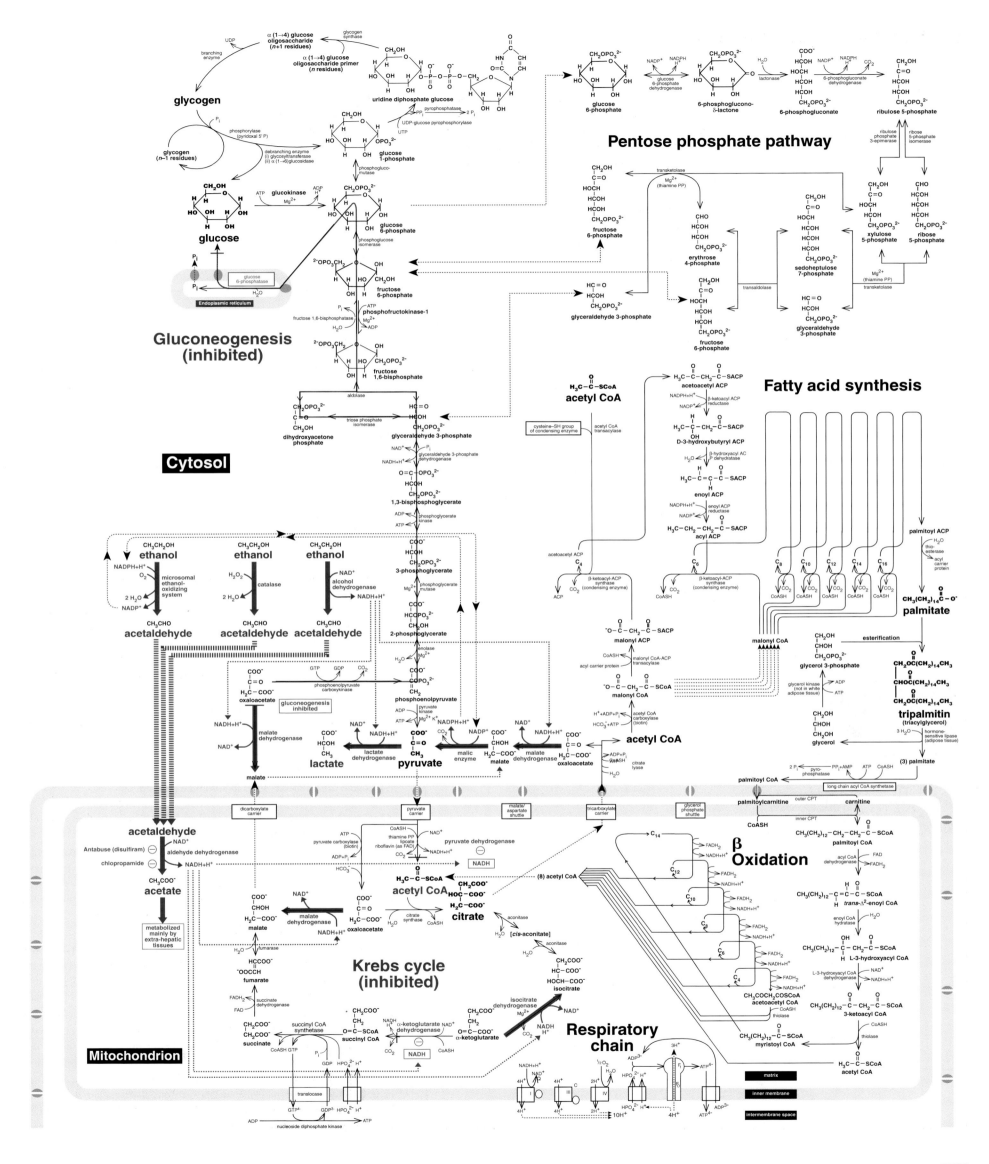

101

Sorbitol, galactitol, glucuronate and xylitol

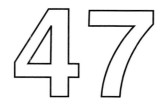

Chart 47.1: Sorbitol, the dietary (exogenous) friend but endogenous foe
Dietary sorbitol as a food sweetener

Sorbitol is a sugar alcohol that is used as a food sweetener in diabetic diets, and has a sweetness value approximately 50% that of sucrose. Patients with diabetes can eat small quantities of sorbitol safely because it is transported relatively slowly across cell membranes, and is absorbed slowly from the intestines.

Endogenously produced sorbitol and cataracts: 'the polyol osmotic theory for the formation of diabetic cataracts'

Although the poor ability of extracellular sorbitol to cross cell membranes favours its use as a sweetener for diabetic food, paradoxically this property can also cause problems. This is because sorbitol produced **endogenously** within cells such as neurons and the optical lens, accumulates within the cell and is metabolized very slowly. Under normal circumstances this is not a problem, since **aldose reductase**, the enzyme that converts glucose to sorbitol, has a K_m for glucose of 70 mmol/l. Hence, it is relatively inactive when the blood glucose concentration is within normal limits of around 3.5–6 mmol/l. However, in uncontrolled diabetes with glucose levels of 25 mmol/l or higher, sorbitol formation occurs at a greater rate, and elevated tissue sorbitol levels have been implicated with certain complications of diabetes such as neuropathy, cataracts and vascular disease. For example, *in vitro* studies have shown that if rabbit lenses are incubated in media containing very high glucose concentrations (35 mmol/l), they accumulate sorbitol. Consequently, the intralenticular osmotic pressure increases causing the lens to swell and become opaque. This can be prevented by aldose reductase inhibitors, such as sorbinil.

Sorbitol catabolism

Sorbitol is metabolized by **sorbitol dehydrogenase** (see Chart 47.1), which is particularly active in liver, to form fructose in a reaction coupled to the formation of NADH. This increases the cytosolic NADH/NAD$^+$ ratio, which both favours the reduction of dihydroxyacetone phosphate to glycerol 3-phosphate and inhibits glycolysis by favouring the reduction of 1,3-bisphosphoglycerate to glyceraldehyde 3-phosphate. Also, experiments with rat lens have demonstrated that, when the aldose reductase pathway is active, the sorbitol formed is metabolized by sorbitol dehydrogenase to form fructose, which is metabolized to **glycerol 3-phosphate**, since glycolysis is inhibited at the glyceraldehyde 3-phosphate dehydrogenase reaction. Finally, because aldose reductase generates NADP$^+$, the pentose phosphate pathway is stimulated.

Chart 47.2: Galactose and galactitol metabolism
Uses of galactose

Galactose is used as a component of cerebrosides and glycoproteins and, during lactation, is used to synthesize lactose. The major dietary source of galactose is lactose in milk. Hydrolysis of lactose by intestinal lactase yields glucose and galactose. Surplus galactose is metabolized to glucose as shown in Chart 47.2.

Inborn errors of galactose metabolism

Classical galactosaemia is caused by deficiency of **galactose 1-phosphate uridyltransferase (Gal-1-PUT)**. The alternative form is **galactokinase** deficiency, but both disorders have similar clinical features. In both conditions dietary galactose cannot be metabolized. Consequently, it accumulates in the blood and enters the cells of the lens, where it is reduced to **galactitol** by **aldose reductase**. It is believed that this can cause cataracts by a mechanism similar to that described for sorbitol.

Chart 47.3: Glucuronate and xylitol metabolism
Glucuronate conjugates with bilirubin, steroids and drug metabolites

Uridine diphosphate glucuronate (UDP glucuronate) is formed by oxidation of **UDP glucose** in the presence of UDP glucose dehydrogenase. Hydrophobic molecules such as bilirubin, steroid hormones and many drugs are conjugated with glucuronate by **UDP glucuronyltransferase** to form a water-soluble glucuronide derivative before excretion by the kidney. In Crigler–Najjar syndrome (Chart 45.1), deficiency of UDP glucuronyltransferase causes increased levels of unconjugated bilirubin, which is bound to albumin, to accumulate in the blood. If the levels exceed the binding capacity of albumin, the unconjugated bilirubin will be taken up by the brain, causing kernicterus.

Glucuronate is the precursor of vitamin C, but not in humans

UDP glucuronate is metabolized to L-gulonate. In most animals (with the notable exception of humans, other primates, guinea-pigs and fruit bats), L-gulonate can be metabolized to ascorbate (vitamin C).

Metabolism of glucuronate and xylitol: the glucuronate/xylulose pathway

UDP glucuronate is metabolized via the ketose **L-xylulose** to **xylitol**. Xylitol is oxidized to D-xylulose, which is phosphorylated to **xylulose 5-phosphate**, which enters the pentose phosphate pathway before joining the glycolytic (or gluconeogenic) pathway.

Inborn error of metabolism: essential pentosuria

This is a very rare benign condition, most frequently found in Jewish people, in which large quantities (up to 4 g per day) of L-xylulose are excreted in the urine. The condition is due to deficiency of **L-xylulose reductase**.

Xylitol in chewing gum prevents dental decay

There has been much interest in the use of xylitol as a sweetener, since it appears to have properties that limit dental caries. Clinical trials indicate that 7–10 g per day of xylitol in chewing gum can provide good resistance to dental decay in children. This cariostatic effect is thought to be due to both its ability to interfere with the metabolism of *Streptococcus mutans* (the organism in plaque responsible for caries) and also its ability to stabilize solutions of calcium phosphate, which favours remineralization of enamel.

Chart 47.2 Galactose and galactitol metabolism.

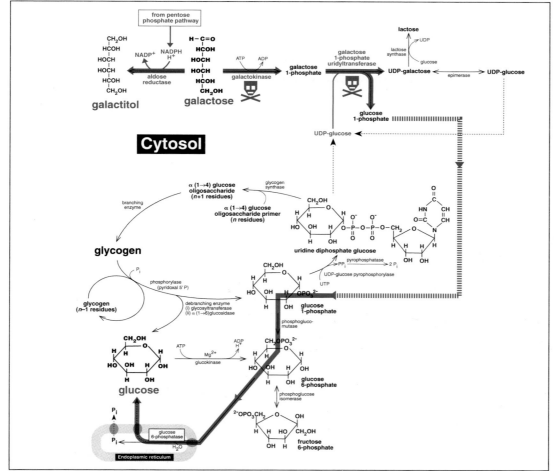

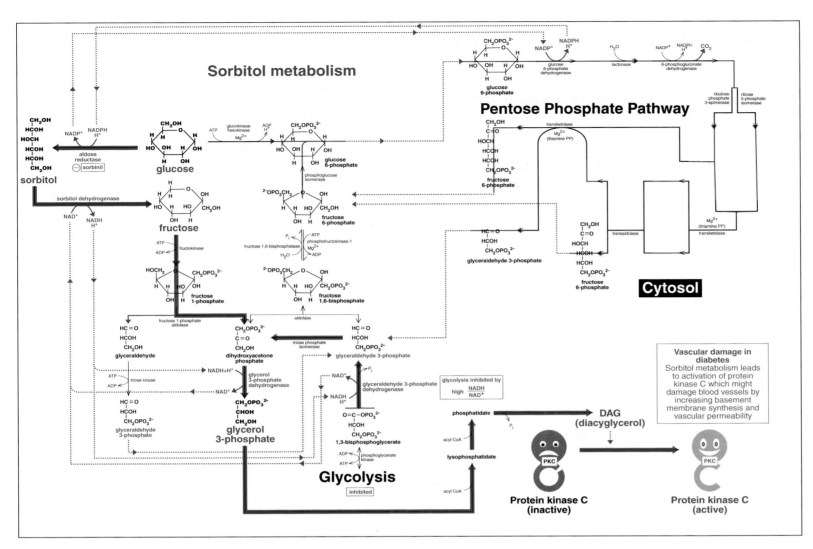

Chart 47.1 Sorbitol metabolism.

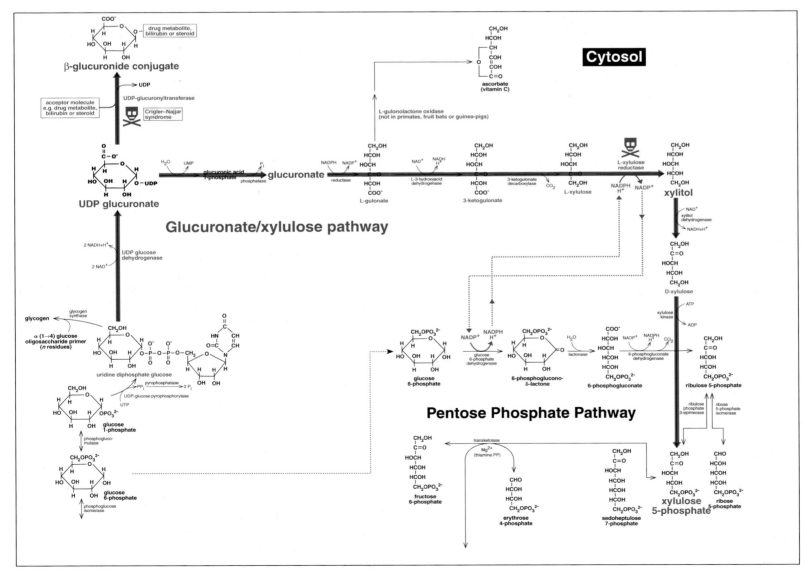

Chart 47.3 Glucuronate and xylitol metabolism.

Fructose metabolism

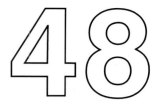

Fructose does not need insulin to enter muscle cells

The average daily intake of fructose in the UK is around 35–50 g, mainly as the disaccharide sucrose. This is hydrolysed by sucrase in the intestinal cells, forming glucose and fructose. Unlike glucose, however, fructose is able to enter muscle cells and adipocytes in the absence of insulin by using the (confusingly named) glucose transporter **GLUT5**. Consequently, it has been suggested that intravenous fructose should be given as an energy source in patients suffering major trauma. However, this practice is not favoured currently because of the risk of lactic acidosis, as described below.

Metabolism of fructose by the liver

Fructose enters the cell via the fructose transporter GLUT5. Then, the liver enzyme **fructokinase** phosphorylates fructose to **fructose 1-phosphate** (see Chart 48.1). This is cleaved by **fructose 1-phosphate aldolase** (aldolase B) to form **dihydroxyacetone** phosphate and **glyceraldehyde**. Glyceraldehyde is then phosphorylated by **triose kinase** to **glyceraldehyde 3-phosphate**. Thus the intermediary metabolites of fructose enter glycolysis as triose phosphates. Their fate now depends on the prevailing metabolic status. However, in the typical circumstances of refeeding after a period of fasting, it is most likely that gluconeogenesis will dominate in the early fed state, so that glycogen and/or glucose will be formed. Alternatively, the substrates could be converted to acetyl CoA and used for fatty acid synthesis.

Metabolism of fructose by muscle

It is likely that the normal dietary quantities of fructose that are presented to the liver in the portal blood will be largely converted to glucose or hepatic glycogen, as described above. Consequently, relatively little fructose will remain for metabolism by muscle. However, if fructose is administered intravenously under experimental conditions, it is metabolized to fructose 6-phosphate by **hexokinase**, since fructokinase is absent from muscle (see Chart 48.2). The subsequent fate of this fructose 6-phosphate will depend on the prevailing nutritional status, which will determine whether it is converted to glycogen or used as a respiratory fuel.

Dangers of intravenous fructose

Fructose is metabolized rapidly in humans, having a half-life of 18 minutes. In fact, it disappears from the circulation twice as rapidly as glucose. Although intravenous fructose was once recommended for use in parenteral nutrition, it was not without risk. These dangers accrue because fructose by-passes the regulatory steps that control glucose catabolism in the following ways:

1 The entry of fructose into muscle uses GLUT5, which is independent of insulin.

2 Intravenous feeding with large quantities of fructose depletes cellular inorganic phosphate (P_i) and lowers the concentration of ATP. Thus phosphofructokinase is deinhibited in muscle, and uncontrolled glycolysis from fructose 6-phosphate proceeds with production of lactic acid.

3 In liver, fructose evades the rate-limiting control mechanism by entering glycolysis as dihydroxyacetone phosphate or glyceraldehyde 3-phosphate, i.e. beyond the regulatory enzyme, phosphofructokinase-1. The consequence of these effects could be that, in anoxic states, such as result from the shock of severe trauma, rapid intravenous infusion of fructose may cause a massive unregulated flux of metabolites through glycolysis. In extreme circumstances this has led to the production of excessive quantities of lactic acid and precipitated fatal lactic acidosis.

Inborn errors of metabolism
Fructokinase deficiency (essential fructosuria)

This benign condition is due to a congenital absence of **fructokinase** and is most commonly found in Jewish families. The deficiency means that ingested fructose is limited to metabolism by the hexokinase route only. Consequently, fructose is metabolized much more slowly than usual, so that the blood concentration rises and fructose appears in the urine. Subjects with essential fructosuria have an entirely normal life expectancy.

Fructose 1-phosphate aldolase deficiency (hereditary fructose intolerance)

This serious condition usually presents when an infant is weaned from breast milk on to fructose-containing food. The response to fructose ingestion is a dramatic onset of vomiting and hypoglycaemia within 15–30 minutes. The disorder is due to a deficiency of **fructose 1-phosphate aldolase (aldolase B)**, which results in a massive accumulation of fructose 1-phosphate in the tissues (see Chart 48.1). This process sequesters intracellular inorganic phosphate, and moreover inhibits both glycogen **phosphorylase** and fructose 1,6-bisphosphate aldolase (**aldolase A**). The resulting inhibition of glucose production by both glycogenolysis and gluconeogenesis causes the severe hypoglycaemia that is such a serious feature of this condition.

Treatment involves simply avoiding dietary fructose. Patients tend to develop a natural aversion to sweet foods and this usually leads to a complete absence of dental caries. If the condition is not diagnosed and treated, the disease is fatal.

Fructose 1,6-bisphosphatase deficiency

This is a disease caused by impaired hepatic gluconeogenesis due to deficiency of this enzyme (see Chart 48.1). It is surprising that, given the strategic importance of fructose 1,6-bisphosphatase in maintaining gluconeogenesis, some patients are relatively unaffected by this disorder. However, in other cases, infants may be hospitalized during the first 6 months of life when the metabolic stress of an infection or fever precipitates hypoglycaemia and lactic acidosis. Although some children with this condition have hepatomegaly and are extremely ill, curiously in other cases this disorder may not be manifested until adult life.

The biochemical pathology results from the stress of trauma or infection provoking a catabolic state in which lipolysis and muscle breakdown combine to produce gluconeogenic amino acids and glycerol. Because gluconeogenesis is inhibited at the fructose 1,6-bisphosphatase reaction, the gluconeogenic metabolites accumulate and form large quantities of lactate. Similarly, ingestion of fructose leads to the formation of lactic acid, precipitating lactic acidosis.

In this condition, glycogenolysis by the liver to release glucose is normal. However, once glycogen is depleted, hypoglycaemia follows due to the failure of gluconeogenesis to maintain glucose homeostasis. These patients must therefore eat frequent meals to maintain normoglycaemia.

Fructose enhances glucose utilization by causing the translocation of glucokinase from the hepatocyte nucleus to the cytosol

Although it has been known for a long time that fructose enhances glucose utilization by the liver, the mechanism has hitherto not been understood. However, recent evidence suggests that an extraordinary and novel control process might be involved. Surprisingly, it appears that in the fasting state, glucokinase is located in the hepatocyte nucleus, where it is bound to the **glucokinase regulatory protein (GKRP)**, which is a 62 kDa protein and functions as a nuclear anchor (see Diagram 48.1). The binding to GKRP is facilitated by fructose 6-phosphate. After feeding, fructose is metabolized rapidly to fructose 1-phosphate, which causes glucokinase to dissociate from the GKRP, enabling the liberated and active glucokinase to diffuse to the cytosol. This effect is caused by very low (0.2 mmol/l) concentrations of fructose 1-phosphate, or high (15 mmol/l) concentrations of glucose.

The advantages of this control mechanism is the subject of speculation. It could be that removal of glucokinase to the nucleus prevents the futile cycling of **glucose → glucose 6-phosphate → glucose** that would occur if both glucokinase and glucose 6-phosphatase were simultaneously active. Also, localization in the nucleus might provide a safe haven for glucokinase from proteolytic attack. Alternatively, the nuclear localization of glucokinase might be important for those genes where transcription is stimulated by an abundance of glucose, such as the lipogenic enzymes: liver L-type pyruvate kinase, fatty acid synthase and stearoyl CoA desaturase.

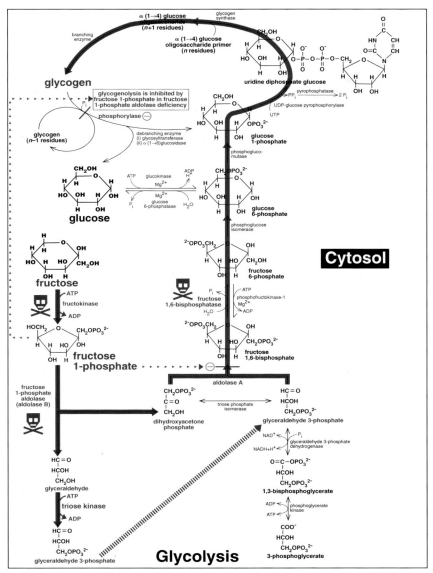

Chart 48.1 Metabolism of fructose to glycogen in liver.

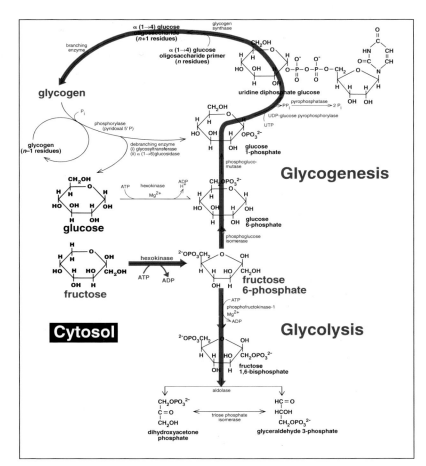

Chart 48.2 Metabolism of fructose in muscle.

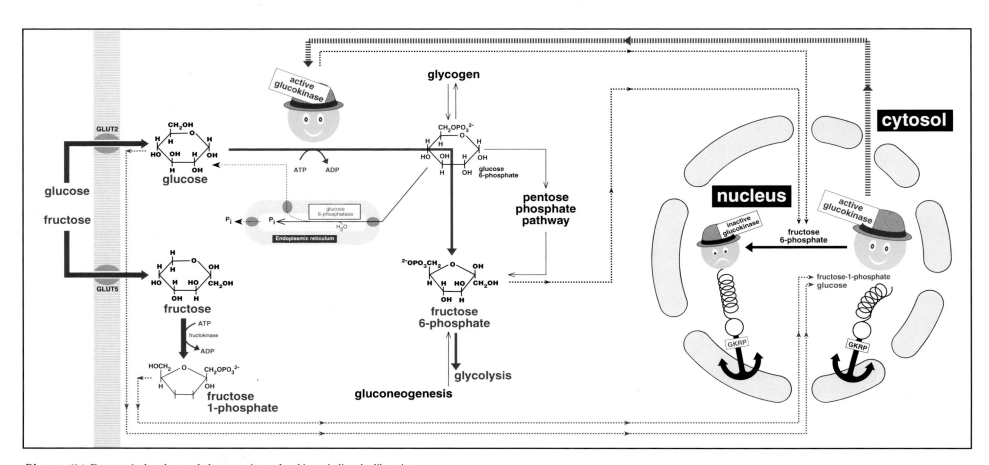

Diagram 48.1 Fructose 1-phosphate and glucose activate glucokinase in liver by liberating it from the nucleus where it is bound to the glucokinase regulating protein (GKRP).

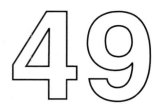

Metabolic mutual dependence

In a splendid example of '*United we stand, divided we fall*' the pathways for **gluconeogenesis**, **β-oxidation**, the **urea cycle**, **ketogenesis** and the **respiratory chain** are mutually dependent (Chart 49.1). The demand for ATP in liver during fasting principally arises from (**i**) the need for ATP by **gluconeogenesis**, which maintains the blood glucose concentration; and (**ii**) the need for ATP by the **urea cycle**, which disposes of nitrogen from amino acids. To generate ATP in the **respiratory chain**, $FADH_2$ and NADH are supplied by **β-oxidation**, which produces acetyl CoA that is deployed for **ketogenesis**. If all the pathways are functioning optimally, all is well. However, if **even one** of these pathways is not operating adequately, this failure might compromise the functioning of **all** the other pathways. Their mutual dependency is summarized in Table 49.1.

Chart 49.1 (below)
The mutual dependency of the metabolic pathways operating in liver in the fasting state. In liver during fasting, gluconeogenesis, ketogenesis, β-oxidation, the respiratory chain and the urea cycle operate as outlined on the chart. Their mutual dependency is based on their need for a supply of cofactors such as ATP, NAD+, FAD, etc.

Reye's syndrome

In 1963, R.D. Reye (pronounced 'rye') described a syndrome characterized by **microvesicular accumulation of fat** in the liver, **cerebral oedema**, **swollen mitochondria**, **hyperammonaemia** and **hypoglycaemia**. Subsequently, it has also been shown to be associated with **increased blood concentrations of free fatty acids** and **amino acids**, such as glutamine, alanine and lysine. The disease occurs in children suffering from a viral infection that has been treated with aspirin (or a combination drug containing aspirin). In what has been declared a 'public health triumph,' by withholding aspirin from children the disease is now very rare. Furthermore, early diagnosis and treatment has dramatically reduced mortality (originally 50%) and neurological damage. The exact pathophysiology is not understood but it is possible that aspirin or its metabolites might inhibit **β-oxidation** in fasting liver (Chart 49.1) and consequently restrict **all the other** dependent pathways as shown in Chart 49.2

Reye-like syndrome

About 30 inborn errors of metabolism have been shown to mimic classical aspirin-induced Reye's syndrome. Although at first glance they may seem many and varied, nearly all of them can be classified into groups causing impaired functioning of either **β-oxidation**, **gluconeogenesis**, **ketogenesis**, the **urea cycle** or the **respiratory chain** (see Chart 49.2). Failure of just **one** of these pathways leads to restriction of them **all** with microvesicular fat accumulation in the liver, hypoglycaemia and hyperammonaemia as in classical Reye's syndrome described above.

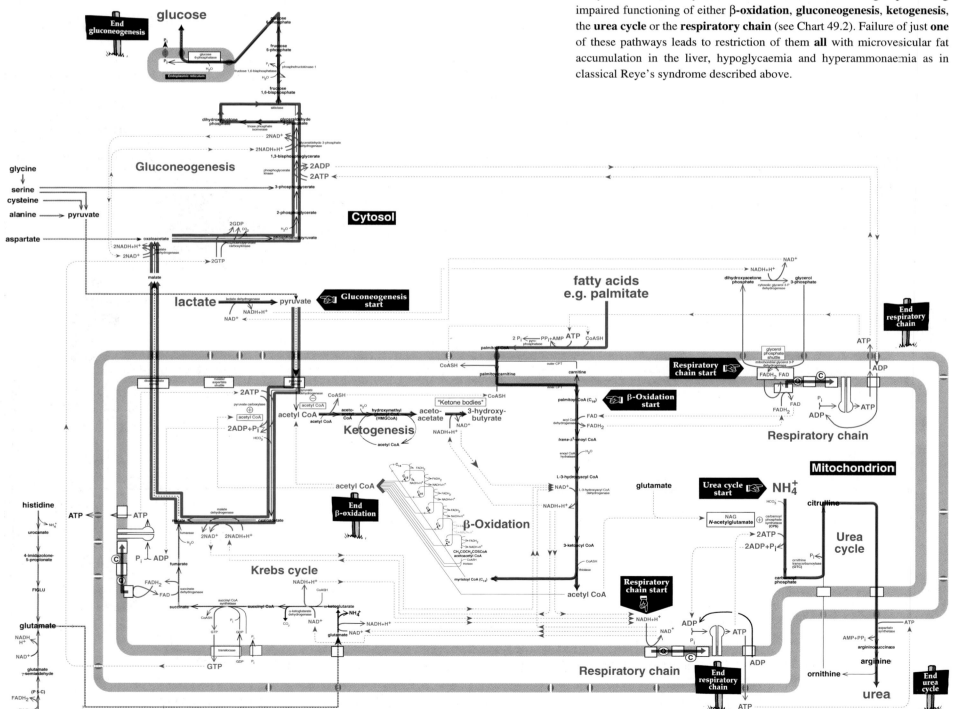

Table 49.1 The mutual interdependence of the metabolic pathways operating in liver during fasting.

Pathway	Substrates or cofactors needed for the pathway to operate during starvation	Function of the pathway	Consequences of pathway malfunction (*Signs characteristic of Reye's syndrome)
Gluconeogenesis (Chapter 23)	• **Carbon source** such as the glycogenic amino acids. • **ATP** from the respiratory chain & GTP from Krebs. • **Acetyl CoA** from β-oxidation activates pyruvate carboxylase.	• **Produces glucose** during fasting which prevents hypoglycaemia.	• **Hypoglycaemia***, which if severe can cause brain damage.
β-Oxidation (Chapters 15 & 29)	• **ATP** for the acyl CoA synthetase reaction is supplied by the respiratory chain. • **FAD** and **NAD+** from the respiratory chain and **NAD+** from ketogenesis. • **CoASH** is supplied by ketogenesis.	• **Produces acetyl CoA** mainly for ketogenesis. • **Acetyl CoA is also used to make NAG**, an allosteric stimulator of the urea cycle, which produces urea. • **FADH₂** and **NADH** are oxidized in the the respiratory chain to form **ATP**.	• **Fatty acids and triacylglycerol (microvesicular fat) accumulate in liver*** because they cannot be oxidized. • **Ketogenesis is impaired, hypoketonaemia***. Impaired production of NAG restricts function of the urea cycle causing neurotoxic **hyperammonaemia***. • **FADH₂** and **NADH** are not available for ATP production by the respiratory chain.
Ketogenesis (Chapter 27)	• **Acetyl CoA** provided by β-oxidation forms the ketone bodies, i.e. acetoacetate and 3-hydroxybutyrate. • **NADH** is supplied by β-oxidation.	• **Ketone bodies** are used by the brain during starvation thus sparing glucose.	• The supply of ketone bodies is decreased so the brain must use glucose as a fuel. But if gluconeogenesis is also impaired, glucose supply is restricted, hence **hypoglycaemia***.
Urea cycle (Chapter 33)	• **ATP** supplied by the respiratory chain. • **NAG** an allosteric stimulator of CPS.	• **Detoxifies ammonia**, which is a waste product of amino acid metabolism.	• **Hyperammonaemia***, which can cause brain damage.
Respiratory chain (Chapter 3)	• **FADH₂** and **NADH** supplied by β-oxidation. • **ADP** and **Pᵢ** supplied by the hydrolysis of ATP in gluconeogenesis and the urea cycle.	• **Produces ATP.** • **Produces FAD and NAD+** which are needed for β-oxidation.	• Because ATP is needed for gluconeogenesis, the urea cycle and β-oxidation, these pathways will be inhibited if ATP production is impaired.

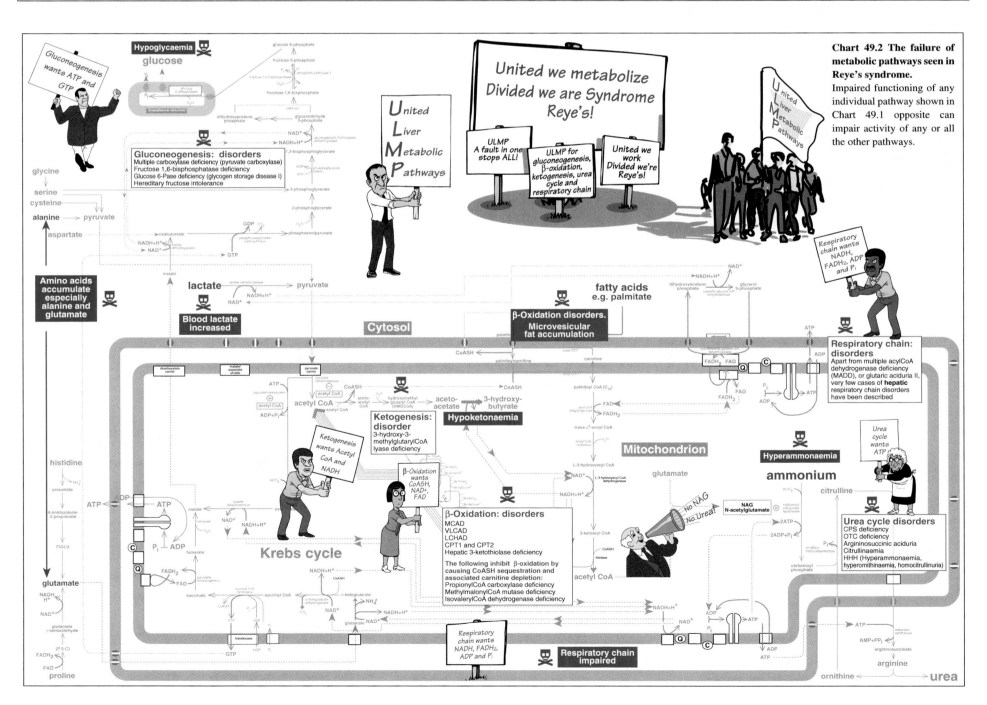

Chart 49.2 The failure of metabolic pathways seen in Reye's syndrome.
Impaired functioning of any individual pathway shown in Chart 49.1 opposite can impair activity of any or all the other pathways.

Diabetes I: insulin-stimulated glucose uptake into cells and glycogen synthesis – signal transduction

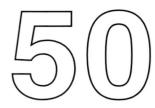

Diagram 50.1 (opposite)
Hypothetical schemes showing how insulin might stimulate glucose uptake and glycogen synthesis.

Although it is commonly known that insulin lowers the blood glucose concentration, in reality insulin has wide-ranging effects not only on metabolism but also on potassium homeostasis, cell volume, cell growth and differentiation. Remarkably, the **multiple effects** of insulin are expressed through a **single type** of insulin receptor. The binding of insulin to its receptor initiates its diverse, or **pleiotropic** effects (Greek *pleion*, more; *tropos*, turn) through a complex signalling system that is not fully understood. Diagram 50.1 summarizes two current hypothetical mechanisms for insulin-stimulated translocation of GLUT4 glucose transporters to plasma membranes to promote glucose uptake, and for insulin-stimulated glycogen synthesis. Both hypotheses involve signalling proteins, some of which are activated or inactivated by reversible protein phosphorylation (Table 50.1).

*NB: It is inherent in scientific progress that aspects of these hypotheses are controversial and they may soon be obsolete as new discoveries are made. Nevertheless, some details **are** withstanding the rigours of experimentation in this very important research that promises exciting new strategies for developing drugs to treat diabetes.*

Insulin-stimulated translocation of GLUT4 to the plasma membrane: CAP/Cbl hypothesis

The proteins participating in the CAP/Cbl hypothesis are listed in Table 50.1 below. The binding of **insulin** to the **insulin receptor** (Diagram 50.1) causes autophosphorylation of the latter, which attracts **associated protein substrate (APS)** to the membrane and causes APS itself to become phosphorylated. Phosphorylated APS attracts **Cbl**, which in turn is phosphorylated. Phosphorylated Cbl associates with **Cbl-associated protein (CAP)**, which binds to **flottilin**, a protein associated with **lipid rafts** in the plasma membrane.

Cbl binds to **Crk**, which is constitutively attached to the GDP/GTP exchange protein **C3G**. Finally, C3G removes GDP from **TC10** and replaces

it with **GTP** thereby activating TC10. This active form of TC10 is thought to induce '**actin comet tails**' on GLUT4-containing vesicles, which propel the vesicles towards the plasma membrane. Upon arrival at the membrane, the **vesicle SNARE** proteins bind to the **target SNARE** complex, which is regulated by interactions with **Munc18c** and/or **synip**. This causes membrane fusion to occur and GLUT4 proteins are inserted into the membrane resulting in uptake of glucose into the cell.

Insulin-stimulated glycogen synthesis and GLUT4 translocation: PDK/PKB hypothesis

This proposes that binding of insulin to its receptor phosphorylates **insulin receptor substrate 1 (IRS-1)** (Diagram 50.1) causing it to attract **p85**, which binds to and activates **phosphatidylinositol-3 kinase (PI-3 kinase)**. This forms **phosphatidylinositol 3,4,5-trisphosphate**, which binds both **protein kinase B (PKB)** and **phosphoinositide-dependent kinase 1 (PDK-1)**, juxtapositioning them in the membrane and enabling PDK-1 to phosphorylate and activate PKB. PKB in turn phosphorylates and inactivates **glycogen synthase kinase 3 (GSK-3)**. Because GSK-3 is constitutively active and inhibits **glycogen synthase**, inactivation of GSK-3 permits glycogen synthesis. PKB also phosphorylates proteins involved in GLUT4 translocation.

References
Alberts B. *et al. The molecular biology of the cell*, 4th edn. N.Y. Garland Science. Compact disc, 25.2, Listeria parasites.

Cohen P. (1999) The Croonian Lecture 1998. *Phil. Trans R Soc London B* **354**, 485–95.

Khan A.H. & Pessin J.E. (2002) Insulin regulation of glucose uptake. *Diabetologia* **45**, 1475–83.

Liczano J.M. & Alessi D. (2002) The insulin signalling pathway. *Curr Biol* **12**, R236–R238.

Table 50.1 The proteins involved in the CAP/Cbl and PDK/PKB pathways for insulin signal transduction.

Icon	Signalling component	Description	Function
	Insulin receptor	A protein tyrosine kinase located in the plasma membrane. Heterotetramer of two 165 kDa α-subunits and two 95 kDa β-subunits linked by disulphide bonds.	Binding of insulin to the α-subunits causes a conformational change stimulating the β-subunit to phosphorylate both itself (autophosphorylation), and IRS-1
	APS (Associated Protein Substrate)	Adaptor protein with pleckstrin homology (PH) and SH2 domains. Member of family of tyrosine kinase adaptor proteins. Interacts with the insulin receptor kinase which stimulates tyrosine 618 phosphorylation of APS	Adaptor protein which facilitates coupling of the insulin receptor to Cbl which enables tyrosine phosphorylation of Cbl by the insulin receptor. APS coupling of Cbl to the insulin receptor causes ubiquitination of the insulin receptor.
	IRS-1 (Insulin Receptor Substrate-1)	Substrate for the insulin receptor. IRS-1 is a 131 kDa cytosolic protein which is **activated** when its 22 tyrosine residues are phosphorylated by the insulin receptor. These phosphorylated tyrosines provide "docking" sites which bind the SH-2 domain proteins. Conversely, IRS-1 is **inactivated** by phosphorylation of serine 307 in rats, or serine 312 in humans.	
SH-2 domain proteins (Src Homology)	(Src: Product of the sarcoma virus, ie **Sarcoma causing protein.**)	SH-2 domain: a polypeptide section of a protein with a high affinity for phosphorylated tyrosine residues.	SH-2 domain proteins function as adaptors and have been described as "molecular velcro"
	Crk /C3G complex (Crk and C3G are constitutively bound)	Crk: A small adaptor protein that links Cbl to C3G.	Crk has a SH2 domain that binds to the tyrosine-phosphorylated Cbl. It also has a SH3 domain which binds to a proline-rich motif C3G
		C3G: A rho-family guanine nucleotide exchange factor	C3G functions as a guanine nucleotide exchange factor and activates TC10
	p85 (regulatory sub-unit of PI-3 kinase)	The 85 kDa protein subunit which regulates PI-3 kinase activity	p85 functions as an adaptor by linking IRS-1 to PI-3 kinase
Signalling proteins: CAP/Cbl pathway for GLUT4 recruitment			
	Lipid raft	Microdomains in the plasma membrane with a distinct lipid and protein content which do not mix with other lipids in the membrane.	Lipid rafts are microdomains in the plasma membrane which contain e.g flotillin, caveolin and palmitoylated proteins.
	Flotillin	A 45 kDa protein present in caveolae (little caves). Named because it floats during sucrose density gradient centrifugation. A component of lipid rafts	Attracts sorbin homology domains
	CAP (Cbl-Associated Protein)	An adaptor protein which joins Cbl to the plasma membrane through the intermediary, flotillin. Has an N-terminal sorbin homology domain and 3 C-terminal Src Homology 3 (SH3) domains	Responsible for targeting tyrosine-phosphorylated Cbl towards membrane. The sorbin homology domain binds to flotillin which is a constituent of lipid rafts. One of the SH3 domains binds Cbl
	Cbl	A member of a family of ubiquitin ligases which down-regulate protein tyrosine kinases by ubiquitination of the receptor prior to degradation. APS phosphorylates tyrosines 371, 700 and 774.	Phosphotyrosine groups on Cbl provide docking sites for Crk/C3G
	TC10	Small GTP binding protein which is expressed in muscle and adipose tissue. An unusual member of the rho-protein family. Insulin stimulation changes TC10 from inactive GDP-bound to active GTP-bound state.	Has major effects on actin especially in adipocytes. Hypothesised that it causes changes in the actin cytoskeleton which are thought to promote GLUT4 translocation to the plasma membrane.
	Actin comet tailing	It was first observed that rapid polymerization/depolymerization of actin could act as a molecular motor in *Listeria monocytogenes* which served to propel the invading bacterium through the viscous cytosol of the host cell. As the actin depolymerizes in the wake of the moving bacterium, it resembles a "comet tail". It is postulated that insulin activates TC10 which induces comet tails on GLUT4-containing vesicles (see time-lapse cinematography of *Listeria* in Alberts *et al.*) which propel them towards the plasma membrane.	
Signalling proteins: PDK/PKB pathway for glycogen synthesis			
	PI-3 kinase (Phosphatidylinositol-3 kinase)	A 110 kDa protein which is active when bound to the SH-2 domain protein, p85. Inhibited by wortmannin.	Phosphorylates phosphatidylinositol 4,5-bisphosphate (PI-4,5-bis P), to form phosphatidylinositol 3,4,5-trisphosphate (PI-3,4,5-tris P).
	PDK-1 (Phosphoinositide Dependent Kinase-1)	A 67 kDa protein which is constitutively active. PI-3,4,5-tris P binds to its PH (Pleckstrin Homology) domain. PDK-1 is bound very tightly to PI-3,4,5 trisP which also binds PKB in juxtaposition it so that PDK-1 can phosphorylate site 1 (threonine 308) of PKB.	
	PKB (Protein Kinase B)	A 60 kDa kinase. Has two phosphorylation sites: site 1 at threonine 308; and site 2 at serine 473. Also named as Akt after a product of the retrovirus AKT8. PI-3,4,5-tris P binds to its PH (Pleckstrin Homology) domain.	PKB is recruited to the plasma membrane by PI 3,4,5-tris P in close proximity to PDK-1 thus enabling (partial) activation by phosphorylation at site 1. Site 2 phosphorylation by PDK-2 causes maximum activity. PKB phosphorylates (inactivates) GSK-3. It is also involved in recruiting the GLUT4, to the plasma membrane.
	GSK-3 (Glycogen Synthase Kinase-3)	A cytosolic, serine/threonine protein kinase with many roles in addition to its function in glycogen metabolism.	GSK-3 phosphorylates and thereby inactivates glycogen synthase. This is prevented by PKB which phosphorylates (inactivates) GSK-3: unusually amongst protein kinases, GSK-3 is constitutively active in resting conditions and serves to suppress signalling pathways.

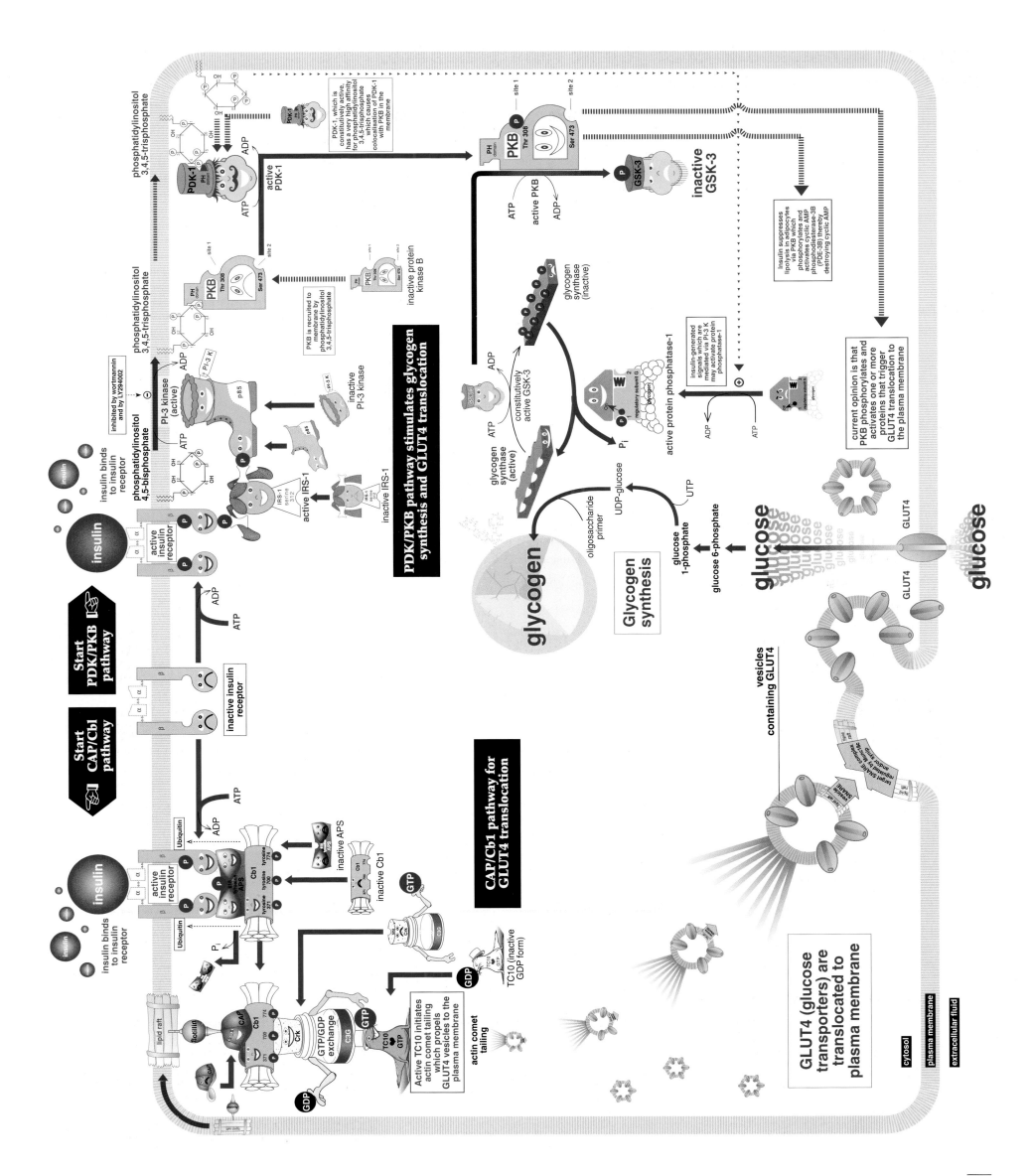

phosphatidylinositol 3,4,5-trisphosphate

PDK-1, which is constitutively active, has a very high affinity for phosphatidylinositol 3,4,5-trisphosphate which causes colocalisation of PDK-1 with PKB in the membrane

active PDK-1

ATP   ADP

PDK-1
PH domain

PKB
PH domain
P
Thr 308
Ser 473

inactive GSK-3

ATP   ADP
active PKB

P
GSK-3

Insulin suppresses lipolysis in adipocytes via PKB which phosphorylates and activates cyclic AMP phosphodiesterase-3B (PDE-3B) thereby destroying cyclic AMP

site 2

PKB
PH domain
Ser 473
Thr 308

site 1

PKB is recruited to membrane by phosphatidylinositol 3,4,5-trisphosphate

PI-3 K
inactive protein kinase B

glycogen synthase (inactive)

ADP
ATP
constitutively active GSK-3

insulin-generated signals which are mediated via PI-3 K may activate protein phosphatase-1

active protein phosphatase-1

ADP
ATP
regulatory subunit G
glycogen

current opinion is that PKB phosphorylates and activates one or more proteins that trigger GLUT4 translocation to the plasma membrane

PDK/PKB pathway stimulates glycogen synthesis and GLUT4 translocation

phosphatidylinositol 3,4,5-trisphosphate

inhibited by wortmannin and by LY294002

PI-3 kinase (active)
ATP   ADP
P   PI-3 K
p85

phosphatidylinositol 4,5-bisphosphate

p85
inactive PI-3 kinase

IRS-1
serine 312
active IRS-1

IRS-1
serine 312
inactive IRS-1

glycogen synthase (active)
P   Pi

Pi

glycogen

UDP-glucose
UTP
oligosaccharide primer
glucose 1-phosphate
glucose 6-phosphate

Glycogen synthesis

insulin
insulin binds to insulin receptor

insulin

α α
β β
active insulin receptor
P   P
P

ATP   ADP

Start PDK/PKB pathway ☞

Start CAP/Cbl pathway ☜

α α
β β
inactive insulin receptor

glucose
glucose
GLUT4
GLUT4

glucose
glucose

GLUT4

CAP/Cbl pathway for GLUT4 translocation

insulin
insulin binds to insulin receptor

insulin

α α
β β
active insulin receptor
P   P
P

ATP   ADP

Ubiquitin

Ubiquitin

SH2 domain
APS
Cb1
tyrosine 774
tyrosine 700
tyrosine 371
inactive APS

Cb1
tyrosine 774
tyrosine 700
tyrosine 371
inactive Cb1

Crk
C3G
GTP

TC10 (inactive GDP form)
GDP
GTP

vesicles containing GLUT4

Pi

lipid raft
flotillin
CAP
Cb1
700   774
371
Crk
C3G
GTP/GDP exchange
TC10
GTP
GTP

GDP

actin comet tailing

Active TC10 initiates actin comet tailing which propels GLUT4 vesicles to the plasma membrane

target SNARE complex required by anchor protein
t-SNARE
v-SNARE
lipid raft

GLUT4 (glucose transporters) are translocated to plasma membrane

cytosol

plasma membrane

extracellular fluid

Diabetes II: metabolic changes in Type 1 diabetes

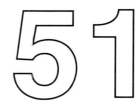

Hyperglycaemia and ketoacidosis in diabetes

In uncontrolled Type 1 (**i**nsulin-**d**ependent **d**iabetes **m**ellitus, IDDM), many metabolic pathways are directed towards the synthesis of glucose and the ketone bodies. This stems from failure of the delicate balance between anabolism and catabolism that is the basis of metabolic homeostasis in healthy adults.

In diabetes, the anabolic state is impaired because insulin is not available to maintain this balance. Consequently, homeostasis is impaired, and catabolism predominates, inducing the following alterations in lipid, protein and carbohydrate metabolism.

Metabolism of triacylglycerol in diabetes

In adipose tissue, insulin prevents triacylglycerol metabolism by inhibiting hormone-sensitive lipase (see Chapter 25). In uncontrolled diabetes, therefore, increased lipolysis results in a 300% enhancement of fatty acid and glycerol mobilization.

1 **Fatty acid metabolism in diabetes.** In the healthy fed state, the fatty acids released by adipose tissue after lipolysis undergo a cyclic process in which they are re-esterified with glycerol 3-phosphate to re-form triacylglycerol (see Chapter 25). In diabetes, this cycle is interrupted due to lack of glycerol 3-phosphate, which is unavailable because it is formed from glucose, which in turn needs insulin to enter the fat cell. Consequently, since re-esterification of the fatty acids is decreased, they are instead released into the blood. Normally fatty acids would be oxidized as a respiratory fuel by most tissues, especially red skeletal muscle. In diabetes, however, surplus fatty acids are transported to the liver where they enter the β-oxidation spiral to form acetyl CoA. In the healthy state, this would usually condense with oxaloacetate for oxidation in Krebs cycle. However, in diabetes, oxaloacetate is removed from the mitochondrion for gluconeogenesis and is in short supply. Consequently, acetyl CoA

molecules combine with each other to form 'the ketone bodies': acetoacetate and D-3-hydroxybutyrate (see Chapter 27). Moreover, in the cytosol, acetyl CoA may be diverted in the direction of cholesterol synthesis, which is often increased in diabetes. In severely uncontrolled IDDM, metabolic regulation is deranged and may be associated with a massive production of acetoacetic acid and D-3-hydroxybutyric acid. In serious cases this overwhelms the pH buffering capacity of the blood causing ketoacidosis.

2 **Glycerol metabolism.** The glycerol released from adipose tissue is phosphorylated in the liver to glycerol 3-phosphate. This is metabolized to glucose, which is released into the blood, contributing to the hyperglycaemia.

Metabolism of protein and amino acids in diabetes

Insulin enhances the uptake of amino acids into muscle from the blood thus favouring protein synthesis. In diabetes, the process is reversed and muscle protein breaks down to form amino acids. Some of these, particularly alanine and glutamine, may be released from muscle and used by the liver for gluconeogenesis (see Chapter 36).

Metabolism of glucose and glycogen in diabetes

Insulin recruits to the plasma membrane the GLUT4 glucose transporters needed for glucose to enter muscle cells and adipocytes. Consequently, in diabetes, glucose accumulates in the extracellular fluids causing hyperglycaemia, while the muscle and fat cells are starved of glucose: a situation described as '*starvation in the midst of plenty*'.

Insulin stimulates glycogen synthesis and increases glucokinase activity. In the absence of insulin, glycogen synthesis ceases and glycogenolysis occurs with glucose being exported from the liver into the blood, once again compounding the hyperglycaemic state.

Diagram 51.1 Metabolic relationship of adipose tissue, muscle and liver in diabetes mellitus. (NB in liver, the bile ducts and canaliculi have been omitted for simplification.)

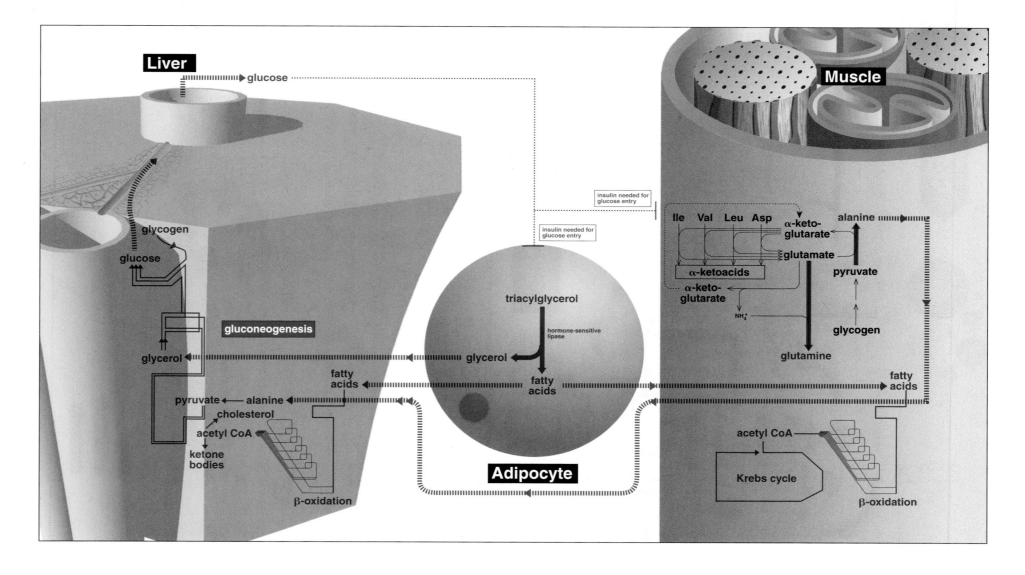

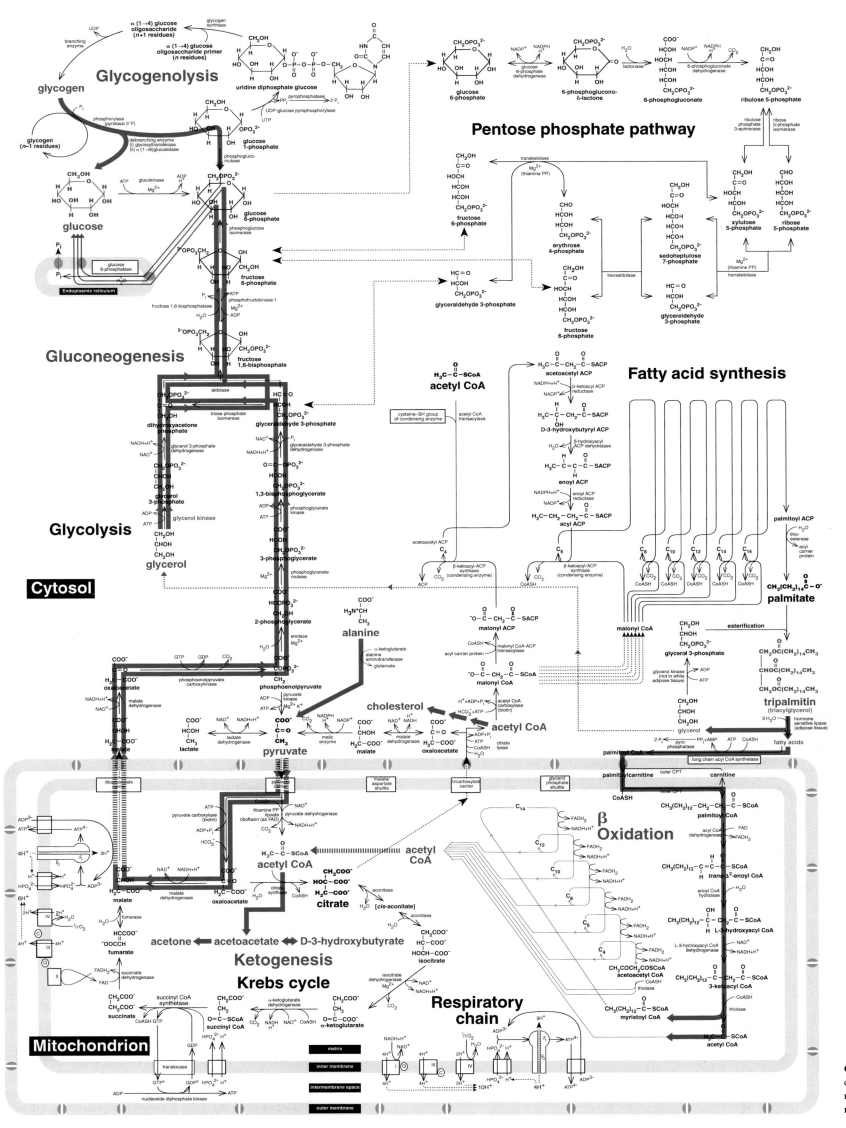

Chart 51.1 An overview of intermediary metabolism in diabetes mellitus.

Diabetes III: Type 1 diabetes, Type 2 diabetes, MODY and pancreatic β-cell metabolism

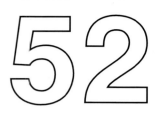

Type 1 diabetes

Type 1 diabetes (previously known as 'juvenile-onset diabetes'), usually occurs before 25 years of age and is the result of β-cell death following viral/autoimmune attack. Consequently, **Type 1 diabetes is characterized by failure of pancreatic β-cells to produce and secrete insulin**. It is treated by insulin replacement therapy and used to be called 'insulin-dependent diabetes mellitus'.

Type 2 diabetes

Patients with Type 2 diabetes (previously known as 'maturity-onset diabetes' or 'non-insulin-dependent diabetes mellitus'), **usually suffer from a combination of defective insulin secretion plus resistance to the action of insulin**. Within the population of patients with Type 2 diabetes, there are probably scores of individual biochemical causes with differing degrees of pathological severity. However, it is postulated that the biochemical cause common to all variants of Type 2 diabetes is that the insulin produced is relatively ineffective. This could be for several reasons, which are the subject of research focused on pancreatic β-cells, skeletal muscle, adipose tissue and liver. For example, secretion of insulin from β-cells is inadequate (insufficient or too slow) following a carbohydrate meal; or (very rarely) the insulin released is structurally abnormal and thus only partially functional. Alternatively, the defects could be in the tissues targeted by insulin, especially skeletal muscle, adipose tissue and the liver. It is possible that the insulin receptor is defective, or that transduction and/or amplification of the insulin signal to intracellular metabolic processes is impaired. Finally it is possible that regulation, by gene expression or phosphorylation, of an enzyme crucial to glucose homeostasis underlies an abnormal response to the insulin signal. In all the above cases, the consequence could be hyperglycaemia and the diabetic state.

MODY (maturity-onset diabetes of the young)

MODY syndrome is an unusual form of diabetes occurring in 1% of diabetic patients. Biochemically, it is characterized by impaired glucose-stimulated insulin secretion by the β-cells resulting in transient hyperglycaemia but without insulin resistance. Whereas Type 2 diabetes is polygenic, MODY is due to a single gene defect with autosomal dominant inheritance. There are six subtypes of MODY. **MODY 2** is a glucose-sensing defect caused by heterozygous mutations of hexokinase. The other subtypes are transcription defects: **MODY 1**, hepatic nuclear factor-4α (HNF-4α); **MODY 3**, hepatic nuclear factor-1α (HNF-1α); **MODY 4**, insulin promoter factor-1 (IPF-1); **MODY 5**, hepatic nuclear factor-1β (HNF-1β); and **MODY 6**, Neuro D1. The transcription factor mutations affect both β-cell development and regulation of genes: for example, HNF-1α and HNF-4α regulate expression of aldolase B, pyruvate kinase, α-ketoglutarate dehydrogenase, GLUT2 and insulin.

The biochemical aetiology of Type 2 diabetes

Glucose homeostasis depends on coordination between the following: (i) the pancreatic β-cell for insulin synthesis, storage and secretion; (ii) skeletal muscle for glucose utilization and, in starvation, provision of amino acids for gluconeogenesis; (iii) adipose tissue for triacylglycerol storage/mobilization; and (iv) the liver for gluconeogenesis, glycogen storage/mobilization, and synthesis of triacylglycerols. An abnormality of any of the above causing hyperglycaemia results in the syndrome of diabetes mellitus.

The inheritance of Type 2 diabetes has been described as 'the geneticist's nightmare'. This is consistent with the multitude of possible biochemical mechanisms for Type 2 diabetes. Undeterred, however, researchers have on the whole shunned the 'shotgun' approach in favour of targeting certain candidate genes, which, in theory if mutated, would result in diabetes. Consequently, in pursuit of abnormalities responsible for the causes of Type 2 diabetes, the products of the 'candidate genes' discussed below have been prioritized for research.

β-Cell metabolism

First, let us consider the **normal** metabolic processes involved in the β-cell, then we can postulate the changes that could contribute to hyperglycaemia and diabetes (see Chart 52.1 opposite). There are two principal mechanisms thought to cause insulin secretion: (i) oxidation of metabolic fuels (especially glucose), which are metabolized **inside the β-cell**; this is known as the 'metabolic fuel hypothesis'; and (ii) potentiation of glucose-stimulated insulin secretion by hormones and other agonists that act on the β-cell **from the outside**.

Metabolic fuel hypothesis for insulin secretion

Oxidative metabolism of glucose by β-cells involves glycolysis, Krebs cycle and the respiratory chain. This increases the intracellular concentration **ratio of ATP to ADP** which provides the metabolic signal for insulin secretion (see Chart 52.1 opposite). This in turn causes the **ATP-sensitive K⁺ channel** in the β-cell plasma membrane to close, resulting in membrane depolarization which activates the **voltage-dependent Ca²⁺ channels** causing calcium influx. The consequential increased concentration of intracellular Ca²⁺ is thought to activate **calmodulin-dependent protein kinase-2** (CaMPK-2), which phosphorylates a protein (or proteins) causing secretion of insulin. **Synaptotagmin** might also act as a Ca²⁺ sensor for the regulation of exocytosis.

Other notable compounds that, when metabolized, stimulate insulin secretion are: **leucine** and, under experimental conditions, **mannose, glyceraldehyde** and **α-ketoisocaproate**.

Another metabolic mechanism for insulin secretion has been proposed. It has been suggested that, when glucose is abundant, it is metabolized to **malonyl CoA** (see Chapter 26), which inhibits transport of acyl molecules by the carnitine shuttle into the mitochondrion for β-oxidation. Instead, the consequent elevation of cytosolic fatty acyl esters, either directly or indirectly – i.e. as lysophosphatidate, phosphatidate or diacylglycerol (DAG) – stimulate secretion of insulin by an unknown mechanism.

Potentiation of glucose-stimulated insulin secretion

Whereas insulin secretion is primarily stimulated by metabolic fuels, such as glucose, this effect can be potentiated by several endocrine and pharmacological agonists that stimulate plasma membrane receptors. For example, **acetylcholine** acts on muscarinic receptors, which activate phospholipase C producing **diacylglycerol**, which activates **protein kinase C** (see Chart 52.1). Also, several hormones that use **cyclic AMP** as an intracellular signal are potentiators of glucose-stimulated insulin secretion, for example, **GIP** (glucose-dependent insulinotrophic polypeptide) and **GLP-1** (glucagon-like peptide-1). They activate **protein kinase A**, which is thought to phosphorylate the same or similar substrates acted on by calmodulin-dependent protein kinase-2 and the other kinases mentioned previously.

Candidate genes that may cause abnormal β-cell metabolism resulting in diabetes

The 'candidate genes' or 'site-specific defects' in β-cell dysfunction are shown in the chart opposite.

Glucose transporter GLUT2. It has been proposed recently that GLUT2 deficiency (both β-cell and liver) may explain the postprandial hyperglycaemia, fasting hypoglycaemia and hepatorenal glycogen accumulation in patients with **Fanconi–Bickel syndrome** (also known as **glycogen storage disease Type XI**).

Glucokinase – 'the pancreatic glucose sensor'. Glucokinase has a low affinity for glucose and so is ideally qualified for the role of glucose sensor. A 30% decrease in β-cell glucokinase activity could increase the blood glucose concentration needed to trigger insulin release from 5 to 6 mmol/l. Heterozygous and homozygous inactivating mutations cause **MODY 2** and **permanent neonatal diabetes mellitus (PNDM)**, respectively. Heterozygous activating mutations cause **persistent hyperinsulinaemic hypoglycaemia of infancy (PHHI)**.

Potassium inwardly rectifying channel 6.2 (Kir6.2). Kir6.2 is part of the β-cell ATP-sensitive channel. Rare mutations cause PHHI, and the common heterozygous E23K (Glu23Lys) polymorphism increases risk for Type 2 diabetes.

Peroxisome proliferator activated receptor-γ (PPAR-γ). PPAR-γ is a transcription factor with a pivotal role in adipocyte differentiation and function. A homozygous disruption of this gene in humans results in severe insulin resistance and Type 2 diabetes. Moreover, a common heterozygous polymorphism P12A (Pro12Ala) is associated with increased risk for Type 2 diabetes.

Chart 52.1 (opposite) Glucose metabolism in pancreatic β-cells causes secretion of insulin.

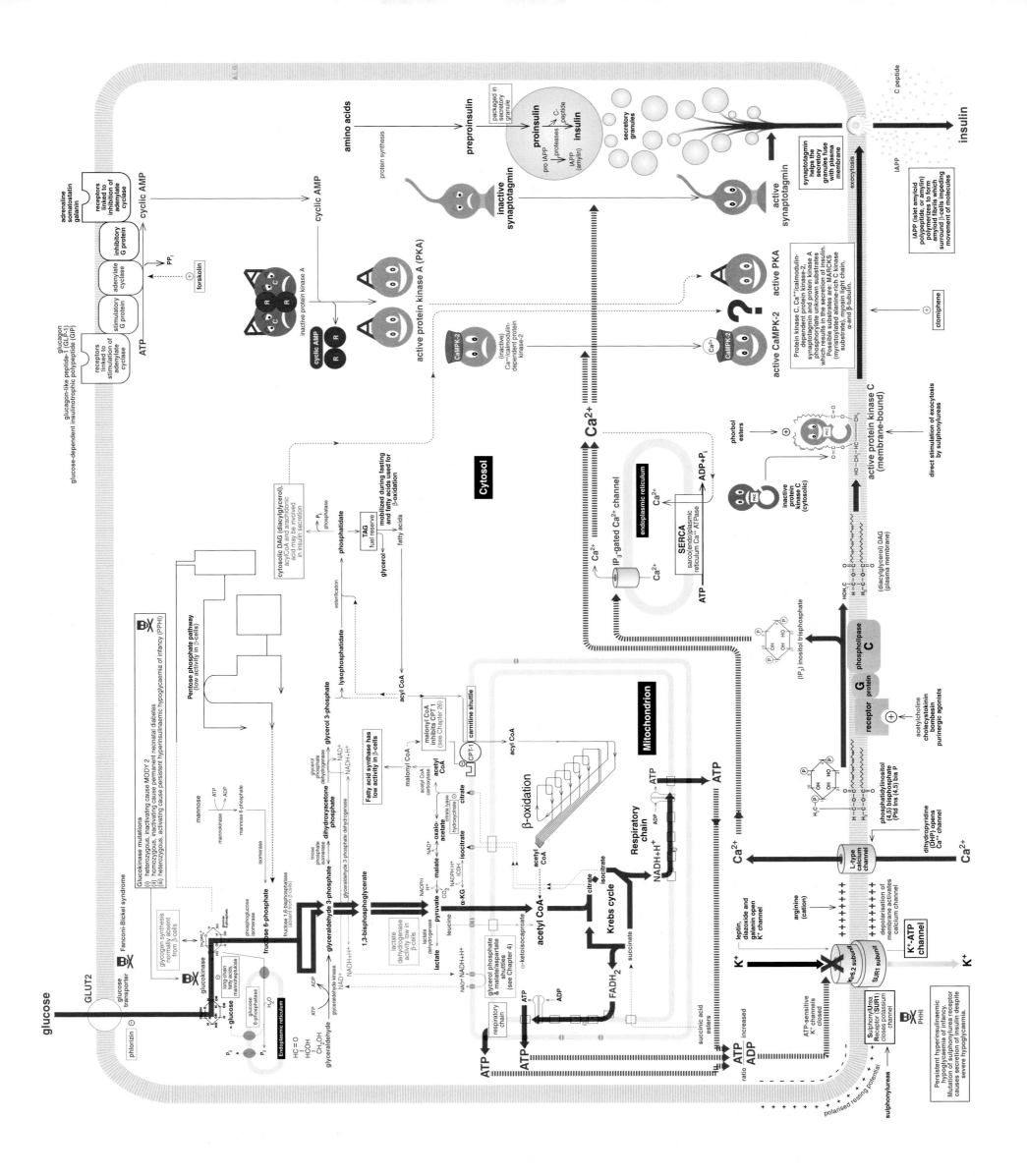

Diabetes IV: Type 2 diabetes and insulin resistance in muscle

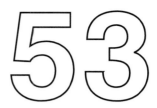

Diagram 53.1 (opposite) Possible sites of insulin resistance in skeletal muscle. The components of the insulin signalling pathway highlighted in red are thought to be prevalent in Type 2 diabetes.

The insulin does not work properly

We have seen how the pathogenesis of some less common forms of the Type 2 diabetes syndrome is due to the impaired ability of the β-cell to produce or secrete insulin (see Chapter 52). The other cause of Type 2 diabetic hyperglycaemia is a blunted response by the target tissues to insulin even though it is secreted by the β-cells in normal or sometimes supranormal amounts in the basal state. Insulin regulates scores of enzymes involved in intermediary metabolism either rapidly, i.e. in minutes, through short-term phosphorylation of enzymes and signalling molecules (see Chapter 50), or alternatively long-term over several hours/days by insulin-regulated gene expression. The diminished ability of insulin to exert its effects on muscle, adipose tissue and liver function is known as **'insulin resistance'**, which is, to widely varying extents, a major feature of Type 2 diabetes. Molecular abnormalities of insulin itself (the 'insulinopathies') or of its receptor, may cause rare forms of diabetes. However, more commonly, there are defects downstream of the receptor in the signalling system or in the enzymes involved in glucose homeostasis.

Insulin resistance in skeletal muscle
Insulin receptor defects
Leprechaunism (Donohue syndrome) and Rabson–Mendenhall syndromes

These are two similar syndromes affecting babies at birth, or neonates, that are caused by mutations to the insulin receptor (Diagram 53.1). Leprechaunism is so called because of the gnome-like appearance of the babies and is usually fatal within one year. This condition restricts binding of insulin at the target tissues and represents the most severe form of insulin resistance. It is characterized by extreme hyperinsulinaemia with concentrations up to 1000 times above normal. Paradoxically, this can cause over-compensation from a hyperglycaemic state after feeding to hypoglycaemia during fasting.

Inactivation of the receptor by dephosphorylation

Normally, binding of insulin to the receptor causes autophosphorylation of tyrosine residues in the β-subunits (see Chapter 50) and initiates insulin signal transduction. Conversely, termination of the insulin signal is by tyrosine dephosphorylation of the β-subunits involving **protein tyrosine phosphatase 1b (PTP 1b)**. Studies on Pima native Americans (an Arizona tribe with 30% of adults having Type 2 diabetes), and other human and animal studies, have shown that increased activity of PTP 1b is associated with diabetes. On the other hand, PTP 1b knockout mice avoid both diabetes and obesity. These and other observations have inspired 34 pharmaceutical companies to produce PTP 1b inhibitors, which promise an exciting new class of antidiabetic drugs for the future.

Post-receptor signalling
Insulin receptor substrate-1 (IRS-1)

Secretion of the cytokine, **tumour necrosis factor-α (TNF-α)**, by adipocytes, is increased in obesity and is thought to cause insulin resistance as follows. Although IRS-1 is **activated** by **tyrosine** phosphorylation, insulin signal transduction is **inhibited** by **serine** phosphorylation (see Diagram 54.2 overleaf). In rats, TNF-α catalyses phosphorylation of serine 307 while in human IRS-1 it is serine 312. This process restricts insulin-stimulated signalling, resulting in the insulin resistance associated with obesity (Diagram 53.1).

Some women with **polycystic ovary syndrome (PCOS)**, also known as Stein–Leventhal syndrome, suffer insulin resistance that may be associated with abnormal forms of IRS-1 causing their hyperglycaemia.

Phosphatidylinositol-3 kinase (PI-3 K)

Because PI-3 K is positioned at a pivotal point in insulin signalling, it has received (together with its p85 subunit) much attention as a candidate for causing hyperglycaemia. Whereas PI-3 K activity is stimulated by insulin, this activity can be reduced by 60% in Type 2 diabetes. Because PI-3 K is a component of the signalling pathway that stimulates the conversion of glucose to glycogen, a defect in this pathway in muscle is likely to cause glycogen breakdown (see Diagram 53.1) producing lactate and alanine, which are used by the liver to form glucose (Diagram 55.1). Also, inhibition of PI-3 K by wortmannin blocks insulin-stimulated GLUT4 translocation.

GLUT4 glucose transporters

The GLUT4 transporter is the gateway for glucose to enter skeletal muscle and adipose tissue. Insulin is the recruiting sergeant that mobilizes the intracellular vesicles containing GLUT4 and inserts them into the plasma membrane (sarcolemma in the case of muscle) (see Diagram 53.1). Studies in patients with Type 2 diabetes suggest there are fewer active GLUT4 molecules compared with controls. However, since vanadate or phenylarsine oxide (**PAO**), which are **protein tyrosine phosphatase inhibitors**, can restore normal glucose transport, the evidence suggests that the fault is in the signalling process (see above) rather than in the GLUT4 molecule itself. Furthermore, when the GLUT4 gene from Type 2 diabetic patients was sequenced, no mutations were detected.

Glycogen synthesis

The amount of glycogen stored at a given time depends on the balance between glycogen production, regulated by glycogen synthase, and glycogen breakdown, which is regulated by phosphorylase. Since the activity of phosphorylase is 50 times that of the synthase, it seems that the glucose molecules in glycogen are straining at the leash awaiting their signal for mobilization to provide energy for the muscle in an adrenaline-driven 'fight or flight' crisis. Evidence suggests that in Type 2 diabetes the insulin signalling system might be defective, permitting glycogen breakdown to exceed glycogen synthesis (see Diagram 53.1). In Type 2 diabetes, therefore, the trend is towards depletion of the glycogen stores despite the prevailing high blood glucose concentrations. Furthermore, some people have abnormal forms of glycogen synthase and suffer hyperglycaemia because they have a restricted ability to convert glucose to glycogen in skeletal muscle.

Glycolysis

Glycolysis (from glucose as opposed to glycogen) is restricted in Type 2 diabetes by the failure to translocate GLUT4 transporters to the sarcolemma despite the prevailing hyperglycaemic state (see Diagram 53.1). Also, the preferential oxidation of fatty acids and (if present) ketone bodies as metabolic fuel, which restricts glycolysis as described below, contributes to the hyperglycaemia (also see glucose/fatty acid cycle, Chapter 24).

Oxidation of fatty acids exacerbates hyperglycaemia

Since the ability of muscle cells to use glucose as fuel is limited by the inability of insulin to function normally in Type 2 diabetes, it is fortunate that muscle is able to use the bountiful supply of fatty acids provided by adipose tissue. Indeed, if muscle has a choice between glucose and fatty acids as a fuel, its preference is the latter. Fatty acids restrict the ability to oxidize glucose thus contributing further to the hyperglycaemic state. This is because acetyl CoA and NADH produced by β-oxidation inhibit pyruvate dehydrogenase thereby diverting the flux of glycolytic metabolites away from Krebs cycle and instead towards synthesis of lactate and alanine. The latter are used by the liver for gluconeogenesis, which exacerbates the hyperglycaemia.

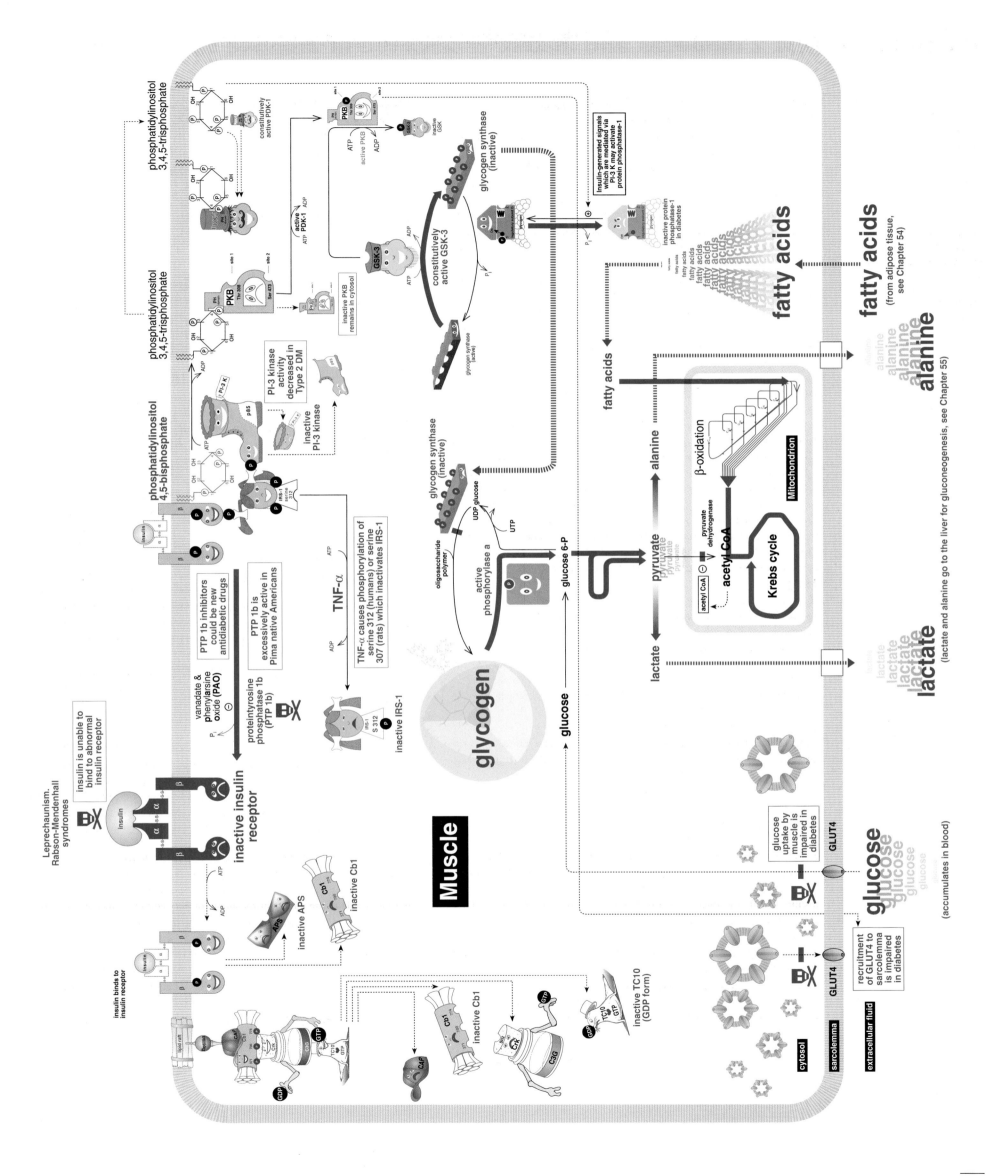

Diabetes V: Type 2 diabetes and insulin resistance in adipose tissue

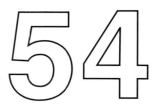

Diagram 54.1 (opposite) Possible sites of insulin resistance in adipose tissue. The components of the pathways highlighted in red are thought to be prevalent in Type 2 diabetes.

Impaired capillary lipoprotein lipase (LPL) activity causes hyperlipidaemia

In the **healthy fed state**, insulin stimulates gene transcription and the synthesis of **lipoprotein lipase** in adipocytes. Lipoprotein lipase is subsequently translocated to the capillaries where it is attached by proteoglycan chains to the endothelium. This response enhances clearance of lipid from both **chylomicrons** and **very-low-density lipoproteins (VLDL)** for storage by adipocytes as **triacylglycerol**. If the insulin signalling mechanism is impaired **in Type 2 diabetes**, this could manifest as deficient insulin-stimulated expression of the lipoprotein lipase gene, causing hyperlipidaemia (see Diagram 54.1).

A signalling fault allows inappropriate lipolysis to occur in the adipocyte

The decreased ability of insulin to cause autophosphorylation of the β-subunit of the insulin receptor in adipocytes from patients with Type 2 diabetes has been reported (see Diagram 54.1). When **insulin is active**, phosphatidylinositol-3 kinase (PI-3 K), through protein kinase B (PKB), stimulates activity of **cyclic AMP phosphodiesterase-3B (PDE-3B)**, which removes cyclic AMP preventing activation of protein kinase A, which, if present, would stimulate **hormone-sensitive lipase (HSL)** (see Chapter 25). It follows that **failure of insulin function** permits cyclic AMP to accumulate and the **activation of HSL** with mobilization of fat reserves (**triacylglycerol**) as glycerol and fatty acids (see Diagram 54.1). Since muscle prefers fatty acids to glucose as a fuel, the fatty acids are preferentially used, which further contributes to the accumulation of glucose in the blood (the glucose-fatty acid cycle, see Chapter 24).

The above suggests a therapeutic strategy to treat Type 2 diabetes, and the HSL inhibitors nicotinic acid (in pharmacological doses) and its analogue, acipimox, have been tested in patients.

A signalling fault results in impaired translocation of glucose transporters

In patients with Type 2 diabetes, fewer GLUT4 glucose transporters are translocated to the plasma membrane in adipose tissue compared with healthy controls (see Diagram 50.1). There is substantial evidence that activation of PI-3 K, phosphoinositide-dependent kinase (PDK) and protein kinase B (PKB) are needed for insulin-stimulated translocation of GLUT4 to the plasma membrane.

Cytokines are important regulators of metabolism in adipose tissue

The cytokines, tumour necrosis factor-α (**TNF-α**) and interleukin-6 (**IL-6**), are made in adipocytes and in obese subjects they are present in the blood in increased concentrations. Cytokines have several effects on metabolism as follows.

Effects of cytokines on lipases in adipose tissue

TNF-α activates hormone-sensitive lipase, which mobilizes fatty acids into the blood (see Diagram 54.1). Furthermore, both TNF-α and IL-6 inhibit lipoprotein lipase, which prevents the clearance of chylomicrons and VLDLs so they accumulate in the blood resulting in hyperlipidaemia.

TNF-α can inhibit the activation of IRS-1 by insulin

TNF-α is associated with obesity, which is a risk factor for Type 2 diabetes. TNF-α inhibits the activation of insulin receptor substrate-1 (IRS-1) by insulin. IRS-1, which is activated when its 22 **tyrosine** residues are phosphorylated by the insulin receptor, is able to propagate the insulin signal, for example, by association with p85 and activation of PI-3 K. However, IRS-1 also has a **serine** residue (serine 307 in rats and serine 312 in humans), which when phosphorylated in response to **TNF-α**, inhibits insulin-stimulated tyrosine phosphorylation of IRS-1 and thus insulin signal transduction (Diagram 54.2).

The hexosamine biosynthesis pathway

Normally only 3% of glucose is metabolized by the hexosamine synthesis pathway (Diagram 54.3), which provides products such as UDP-*N*-acetylglucosamine, UDP-*N*-acetylgalactosamine and sialic acid. However, in diabetes, flux through this pathway is increased and, since 1991, evidence has accumulated which suggests that the increased production of these products can cause insulin resistance. The regulatory enzyme for this pathway is **glutamine:fructose 6-phosphate amidotransferase (GFAT)**.

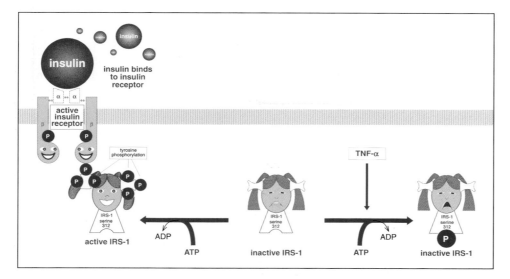

Diagram 54.2 Regulation of insulin receptor substrate (IRS-1) activity.
Phosphorylation of tyrosine sites by the insulin receptor activates IRS-1.
Phosphorylation by TNF-α of serine 312 (human) or serine 307 (rat)
inhibits tyrosine phosphorylation and prevents activation of IRS-1.

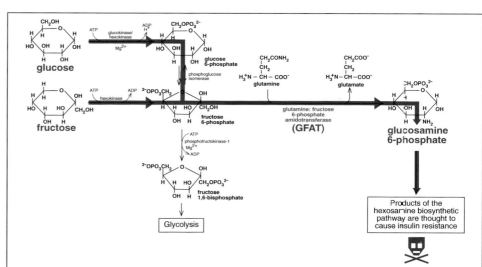

Diagram 54.3 The hexosamine biosynthesis pathway.

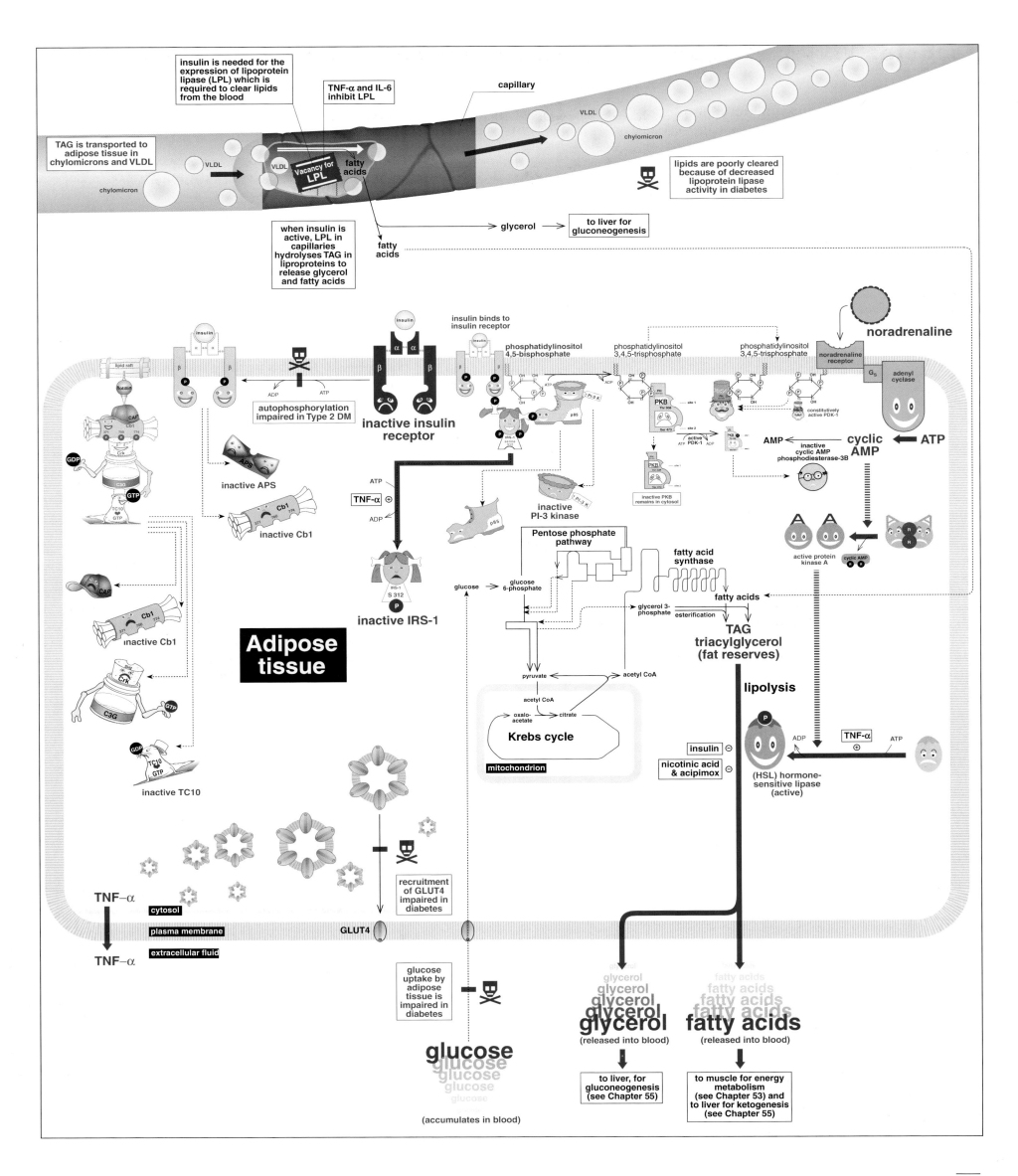

Diabetes VI: Type 2 diabetes and insulin resistance in liver

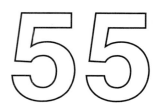

55

Diagram 55.1 (opposite) Metabolic pathways and possible sites of insulin resistance in liver in Type 2 diabetes. When insulin action fails, the signalling proteins are in the state shown in red. In particular, insulin is unable to activate cyclic AMP phosphodiesterase-3 and so cAMP accumulates. This enables the effects of the counter-regulatory hormone glucagon to dominate and the pathways shown in red operate.

Insulin signalling

Insulin **stimulates** transcription of certain genes involved in glucose metabolism and lipogenesis, including genes encoding glucokinase, glyceraldehyde 3-phosphate dehydrogenase, pyruvate kinase, malic enzyme, acetyl CoA carboxylase and fatty acid synthase. Conversely, insulin **inhibits** transcription of the gluconeogenic genes encoding phosphoenolpyruvate-carboxykinase (PEPCK), fructose 1,6-bisphosphatase and glucose 6-phosphatase. Consequently, defects in the signalling mechanisms, e.g. by the PDK/PKB pathway (see Chapter 51), could cause hyperglycaemia either by failure to stimulate disposal of dietary glucose as glycogen or triacylglycerol, or by the inability to inhibit hepatic glucose output (Diagram 55.1).

NB: In liver, unlike muscle, no evidence has been found for regulation of the regulatory subunits of protein phosphatase-1 by phosphorylation/ dephosphorylation. Instead, as shown in Diagram 55.1, phosphorylase a binds to an inhibitory binding site on the regulatory subunit and blocks phosphatase activity.

Hyperlipidaemia

As mentioned in Chapter 54, insulin stimulates phosphodiesterase-3B (PDE-3B), which degrades cyclic AMP and suppresses activity of hormone-sensitive lipase in adipose tissue. Consequently, if this supression fails in Type 2 diabetes, fatty acids will be mobilized from adipose tissue and delivered to the liver. Here they will be esterified to triacylglycerol and secreted as very-low-density lipoproteins (VLDL) causing the hyperlipidaemia frequently seen in Type 2 diabetes. Fatty acids are also metabolized by β-oxidation to form acetyl CoA, which is used for ketogenesis.

Increased hepatic glucose output by liver

As shown in Diagram 55.1, in Type 2 diabetes the liver is presented with an abundance of gluconeogenic substrates, notably **lactate** from skeletal muscle and red blood cells (Chapter 8), **alanine** from muscle (Chapter 36), and **glycerol** from adipose tissue (Chapter 25). The ATP for gluconeogenesis is provided by β-oxidation of fatty acids, the latter being in abundant supply because of the inappropriately high rate of lipolysis in adipocytes as mentioned above. Consequently, an abundance of acetyl CoA is produced, which both inhibits pyruvate dehydrogenase while stimulating pyruvate carboxylase, a regulatory enzyme for gluconeogenesis.

The next flux-regulating step involves PEPCK, which is regulated at the level of DNA transcription. Cyclic AMP mediates the production of PEPCK, whereas insulin inhibits its production. In Type 2 diabetes where there is diminished repression by insulin, PEPCK will be produced, favouring gluconeogenesis.

Hypothesis for the pathogenesis of Type 2 diabetes

Diagram 55.2 illustrates current opinion on the interplay between genetic and lifestyle influences that interact initially to cause mild hyperglycaemia. However, as the years pass, a vicious cycle of ever-increasing hyperglycaemia insidiously contributes to glucose toxicity, eventually manifesting as clinical Type 2 diabetes.

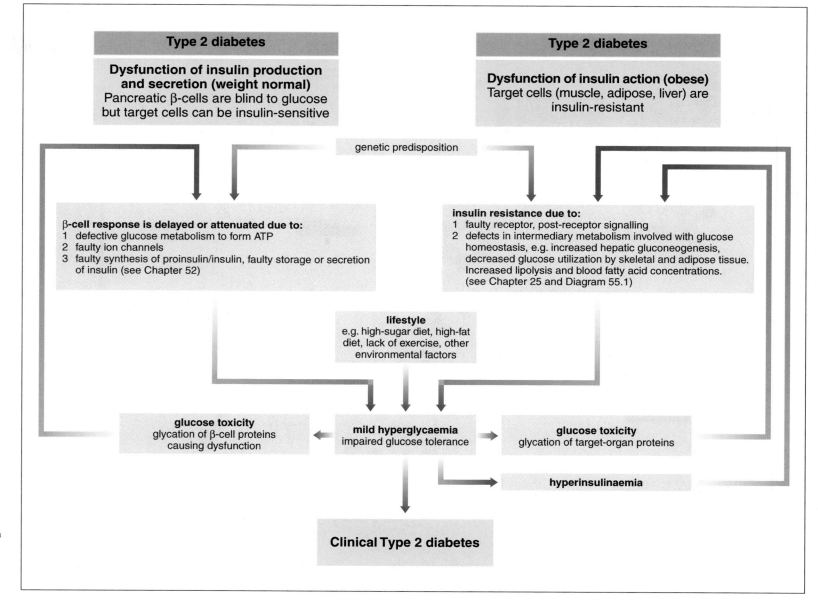

Diagram 55.2 Interplay between genetic and lifestyle influences: a hypothesis for the early stages in the pathogenesis of Type 2 diabetes.

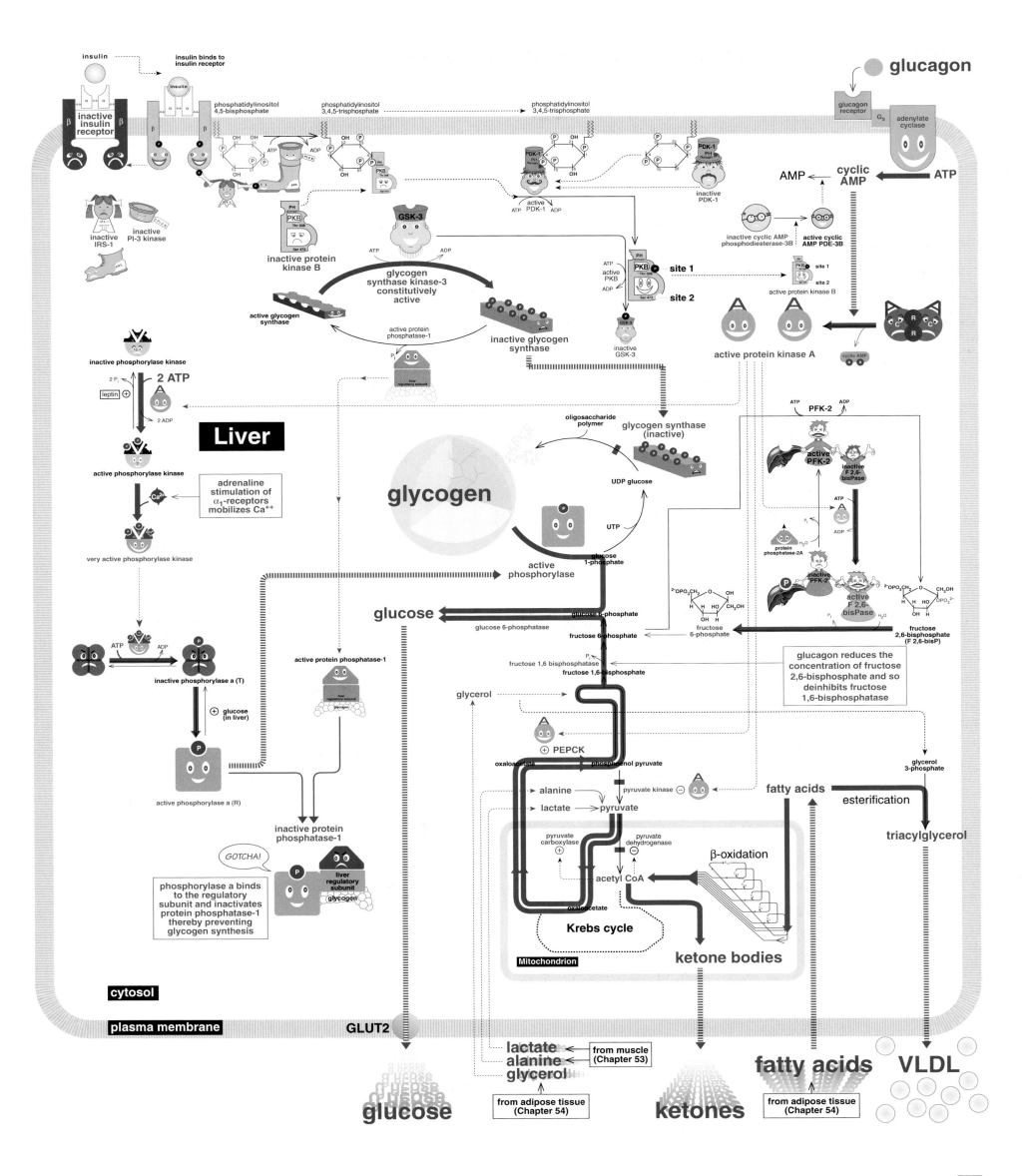

Index

124

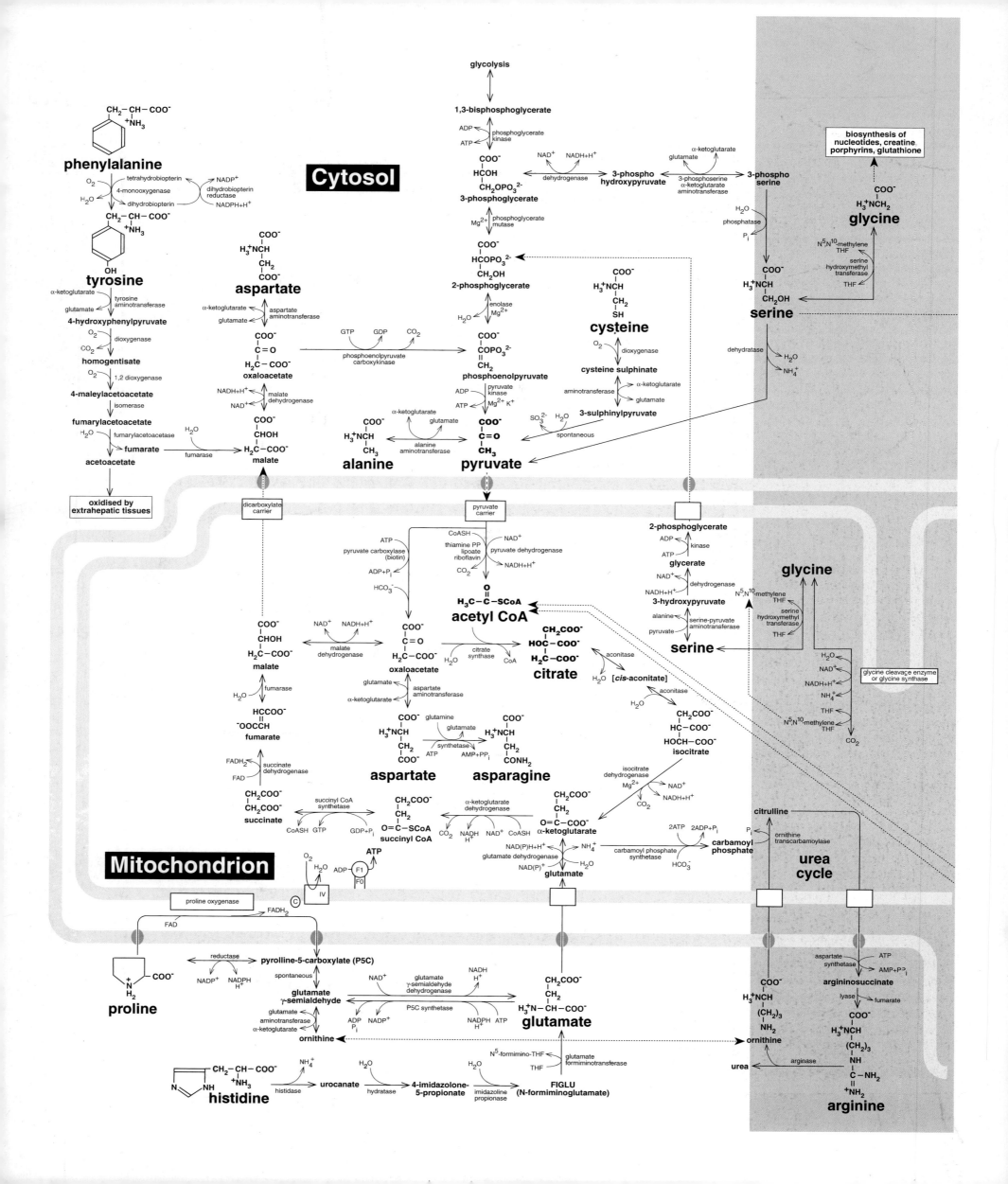